Transforming the Patient Experience

William T. Choctaw, MD

Transforming the Patient Experience

A New Paradigm for Hospital and Physician Leadership

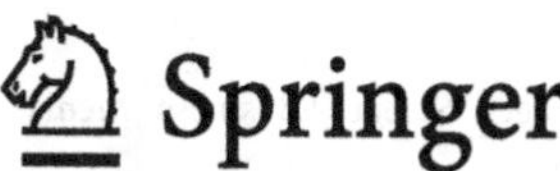

William T. Choctaw, MD
Chief Transformation Officer
Citrus Valley Health Partners
Covina, CA, USA

ISBN 978-3-319-16927-9 ISBN 978-3-319-16928-6 (eBook)
DOI 10.1007/978-3-319-16928-6

Library of Congress Control Number: 2015935275

Springer Cham Heidelberg New York Dordrecht London

Printed on acid-free paper

Springer International Publishing AG Switzerland is part of Springer Science+Business Media (www.springer.com)

Foreword

This story will take you on a journey. A journey through transformational change. Change that was made by fearless and relentless leaders. Leaders who didn't settle for "good enough," but wanted a health care system that did what was right, every time with a singular, shared focus to provide the best and safest patient experience. It is a compelling journey to transform a culture.

To have a transformational change, by definition, one has to change a culture. A culture is defined as an organization's behavior and belief system. There is no easy way to change an organization's culture, especially an ingrained culture of complacency, as was Citrus Valley Health Partners (CVHP) when I arrived in 2008.

Citrus Valley Health Partners, a three hospital system with an inpatient hospice and an active home health agency, had a culture that I perceived as a culture of inertia—don't challenge the status quo, don't rock the boat, let's just keep things afloat. The culture was not transparent, nor visionary. It wasn't concerned about patient care and was okay with being "good enough."

By contrast, today, the culture at Citrus Valley Health Partners is about excelling in delivering the best patient experience and the highest quality of care and outcomes. We have defined our culture by putting safety first and even edited our mission statement to include the word "safe." We have embraced change management and Lean Six Sigma techniques to eliminate waste and improve processes in nearly everything we do. Our pursuit is for zero harm, always, and to become a highly reliable organization. We haven't reached our destination just yet, but the journey thus far has led to an incredible turnaround.

I was asked to join CVHP as its new President and CEO in the fall of 2008. The job specifications were typical in most regard, yet there was an underlying tone that the search committee wanted a new vision for the organization. This committee comprised Board members and physician leaders who knew the organization was in trouble and needed a visionary leader. The competencies, attributes, and deliverables required for this new role are cited below, verbatim, from the search firm's candidate profile:

1. Assure that CVHP's operational performance is "best in class" in the areas of economics, clinical quality, patient safety, and customer satisfaction.
2. Assure that an organization-wide culture exists that emphasizes service excellence and quality care in the delivery of health care services.
3. Assure that the management team is of the highest professional caliber and that a culture exists which encourages optimal individual performance/accountability in a collaborative and harmonious fashion.
4. Develop and implement new and creative approaches to optimizing CVHP's position in the marketplace, meeting community needs, while enhancing the financial strength and reputation of CVHP as a provider of choice.
5. Is skilled at getting individuals, teams, and an entire organization to perform at a higher level and to embrace change.
6. Attacks everything with drive and energy with an eye on the bottom line; not afraid to initiate action before all the facts are known.

It was clear the search committee was looking for a change agent. What struck me as most compelling was one of their final specifications under Leadership Characteristics:

A LEADER who fearlessly takes on all issues, challenges, and people; comfortably confronts and works through conflict; delivers negative feedback and messages without hesitation; deals promptly and fairly with problem performers; lets everyone know where they stand; thrives in crisis and is energized by tough challenges; not afraid to make negative decisions and take tough action; challenges the status quo

This challenge was for me. I knew I could help with the turnaround efforts. There was so much to be done and so much to discover. I distinctly remember one of my first insights into the culture of inertia at CVHP. It was my first time attending the Quality and Performance Improvement Committee (QPIC), a standing committee reporting to the Board. It comprised well-intended clinicians, including prominent physicians and members of the senior management team and, of course, the staff of the Performance Improvement Department.

I listened intently. I have been a student of health care quality and patient satisfaction for over two decades. I have read prolifically on quality and the patient experience and proudly display my text book from the late 1970s written by Dr. Donabedian, the founding father of quality. I also have a personally autographed book by W. Edwards Deming and have had the opportunity to visit Quint Studer, one of the most notable consultants and authors on the patient experience, on many occasions. However, what I realized at the QPIC meeting that day was that they were not following the well-researched nor thoughtful insights of these notable authors. Instead, the presentation of data actually lacked information and, more troubling, provided an almost covert plan to ignore the brutal facts. Quality of care numbers around perfect care were cited, numbers like 84.7 % for Acute Myocardial Infarction and 85.8 % for Congestive Heart Failure—dismal percentages, indeed. It was disappointing that so many of the leaders in the room were satisfied with what appeared to be a "B" average. In addition, patient satisfaction, as measured by Press Ganey, was in the mid-1980s. What was not either understood or purposefully not presented was the relative performance of these metrics. CVHP was in the lowest decile of performance on a comparative basis to both California and hospitals nationwide.

There were many steps along this journey, but I needed to start with my management team. I had to ask my management team to change or I needed to change my management team. In fact, some members did change and I changed some managers. As new leaders arrived and others were discovered within our walls, I had the opportunity to meet an affable, respected, and passionate leader within our medical staff. He is the author of this book and the change agent who co-led this journey with me, William J. Choctaw. M.D., J.D. Dr. Choctaw had been a medical staff leader with CVHP for many decades. He knew the challenges, obstacles and, more importantly, the potential for turnaround and greatness. He and I met frequently and developed a plan. We started by appointing motivated physician and management leaders to form the Transforming the Patient Experience Team. Each member of this team challenged each other to look in the mirror first, hold themselves accountable for their shortcomings and be honest. Once we could see how we must transform ourselves to become better leaders, we can continue to our journey to transform other leaders, physicians, and our culture. The journey has exponentially evolved since its humble beginning 5 years ago. Dr. Choctaw has since appointed more that 50 of his physician colleagues to become mentor coaches seeking transformational change in the behaviors and beliefs of members of the medical staffs.

Today, through the efforts of Dr. Choctaw and the many that stand alongside him, we have a culture that aspires to eliminate harm. The use of the Robust Process Improvement methods of Lean and Six Sigma that improve processes, eliminates waste, and reduces harm have already shown improvements. Our "all cause 30-day heart failure readmission rate" has decreased to 16.7 %; surgical site infections have decreased from 22 in 2013 to 10 in 2014 and they continue to drop. Our hand-off communication defect rate dropped to 25 % from 38 % and our left without being seen rate for one or emergency departments decreased to only 1.5 %. Improvements are being made and will continue as we remain committed to our journey.

Cultural transformative also means we must engage employees and be transparent, always, in what we do and what we say. Our employees agree and have shown us that they are highly engaged through our last employee survey. Our physicians are also more engaged, with the establishment of a physician owned and governed IPA with over 200 physicians participating. Our transformative turnaround has caught the attention of organizations around the country. We have received accolades from the likes of The Joint Commission and Cleverly and Associates. We also serve as a national Blueprint for our quality, financial, and cultural turnaround through VHA. We were featured in Forbes magazine as a model for change management. We have meritorious outcomes as recognized by the American College of Surgeons through the National Surgical Quality Improvement Project. We have gone from an organization that could barely meet its bond covenants of 60 days of cash on hand to an organization that projects 250 days of cash on hand by the end of 2015. Remarkably, our bond rating went from BB (junk bonds) in 2008, to BBB- in 2014 to an astounding triple upgrade in 2015 to bring us to A- rating. In addition, we are now in the top third of all hospitals in terms of patient experience and employee engagement.

With the right culture and the right people, we have also propelled our services. A few examples include: our Center of Excellence in robotic surgery; the only CARF accredited acute rehab unit in the region; COEMIG accredited minimally invasive GYN surgery—one of only 100 in the world; a Certified Primary Stroke Center; on the pathway to a Blue Distinction Orthopedic program; poster child, literally for the County, for door to balloon times and mortality rates for our heart center; a Level IIIB Neonatal unit; a Certified Diabetes inpatient unit; one of the only freestanding Hospice hospitals in the country.

Success has also allowed us to reinvest within our walls and in our community—building community clinics, acquiring a freestanding outpatient surgery center, expanding emergency rooms, our outpatient surgery unit, refurbishing existing lobbies, rooms, and conference centers, investing in state-of-the-art equipment such as Hybrid OR and 3T MRI and in investing in our team by listening to their needs, such as the need for more staffing, and making it happen.

Our story continues. Our journey continues. There are many improvements that still need to be made, but we are well on our way. Throughout this journey—through the challenges, the successes, the disappointments, the wins, the do-overs, and the learnings, what remained consistent was the steadfast commitment and vision of my colleague and friend, Dr. Choctaw. It is not often in life that so many obstacles can present themselves concurrently. It is also not often in life that you find just the right partner to heed these challenges in tandem. This story of our journey is also a story of friendship and true collaboration. I have learned a lot from Bill. He is an astute teacher and visionary. I know his journey, his story, and his teachings will help guide you in creating your story.

Citrus Valley Health Partners
Covina, CA, USA

Rob H. Curry

Preface

This is a story about the combined journey of two healthcare leaders: a hospital CEO and a general surgeon physician champion. It's about how two leaders, who are philosophically in alignment, though from different extremes of the health-provider system, were able to initiate a transformation of the patient experience at a large multi-hospital system. The essence of transformation is teamwork and the least common denominator team is a team of two. The effectiveness of this nuclear team is based on the strength of the working relationship, dependent on mutual respect, mutual trust, and good communication.

The principle of patient centricity to transform the patient experience has fundamentally changed the delivery of healthcare as we know it. Previously, the patient care culture of hospital administration and medical staff leadership were separate, but peacefully coexisted in a calm and genteel medical world. Today, the healthcare world is chaotic and turbulent, while requiring the creation of a single culture with zero harm and higher quality. A new paradigm is necessary to provide quality patient care effectively with high patient satisfaction at a reasonable cost. This new paradigm requires an increased role for physician champions leaders as a third way of medical staff leadership outside of traditionally elected medical staff representatives. The new paradigm requires complete physician integration with the executive management team at multiple levels, in a healthcare delivery system.

Our approach to transform the patient experience is a journey, not a destination. Much work has been done on transforming organizations by John Kotter in business and Quint Studer in hospitals. In the coming pages, I relate what solutions we have found effective for our organization. There is no one silver bullet approach to transform the patient experience but a variety of ways found effective through the prism of time. In the following pages, I share our approach. This book is for all leaders involved in quality and safe patient care, whether in the clinical or management area.

Covina, CA William T. Choctaw, M.D.

Preface

Acknowledgements

I would like to express my deepest gratitude to Rob Curry, President and CEO of Citrus Valley Health Partners. Rob gave me the most precious gift, the gift of "opportunity" by selecting me to be a member of his executive management team. This opportunity has given me an unprecedented scope and perspective on patient-centered care. I am thankful to the entire CVHP family for its encouragement and support.

I am grateful to Anne Marie Benedecto, Klaus Nether, Brian Patterson, Jan Kendrick and Dawn Albee from the Joint Commission Center for Transforming Healthcare for teaching me Robust Process Improvement and Lean Six Sigma principles and tools. I am thankful to my Process Excellence team at CVHP; Denise Ronquillo, Nena LaScala, and Linda Morey for helping me implement many of the Lean Six Sigma principles at our hospitals.

Finally, I thank Lorena, my loving wife, for her suggestions, intelligence, encouragement, and compassionate commitment to bring this manuscript to life.

Acknowledgement

Contents

About the Author

Dr. William Choctaw has been the Chief Transformation Officer (CTO) of Citrus Valley Health Partners since May 2014. Prior to being appointed as CTO, he has served as a member of the medical executive committee at Citrus Valley Medical Center for 10 consecutive years. During that time, he held many medical staff leadership positions, including Chief of Staff and Chief of Surgery. As CTO, he leads the Process Excellence department and is responsible for the implementation of Robust Process Improvement/Lean Six Sigma (RPI/LSS) as part of an ongoing system-wide initiative to dramatically improve the efficiency of hospital internal operations, to increase patient satisfaction, and to ensure that patient care at CVHP is consistently excellent and safe. He is certified Lean Six Sigma green belt and will receive his black belt certification this year.

Dr. Choctaw is a graduate of Yale University School of Medicine. He also has earned a Law Degree from Western University College of Law. He is a member of the Clinical Faculty at University of Southern California School of Medicine. Dr. Choctaw continues to practice general surgery in Covina California.

Chapter 1
Change Is Inevitable

Change is the only constant.
Heraclitus

It has been said that the only constant in life is change. It is this event inevitability that is frequently the source of anxiety in healthcare today. This fact is true for physicians, hospital executives and patients. The relationship one has with change will dictate belief systems and subsequent actions and results. Therefore, it is imperative that change management be a significant component of any attempt to lead a team.

Transformation is fundamental and irreversible change. The essence of transforming any organization is the result of change management process. John Kotter, Harvard Business Review, notes there are eight steps to transformative change. They are:

1. Establishing a sense of urgency.
2. Forming a powerful Guiding Coalition.
3. Creating a Vision
4. Communicating the Vision.
5. Empowering others to act on the Vision.
6. Planning for and creating short-term wins.
7. Consolidating Improvements and producing more Change.
8. Institutionalize New Approaches

Arguably, we are experiencing the greatest healthcare transformation in our nation's history. The effects of healthcare reform, pro or con, will not depend on words used by politicians. The effect will depend on the definition of those words implemented from the healthcare dictionary by all of us. At Citrus Valley Medical Center, we formed a Transforming the Patient Experience Committee based on the principle that patients have a "fundamental right" to quality care. Quality care is not a privilege but a right bestowed upon all humanity. We have subsequently re-committed to the importance of patient safety.

The Transformation the Patient Experience (TPE) committee started with 22 members who looked in the mirror and committed to positively transform the patient's experience at CVHP. We made this commitment because we believe all our patients are equal and should be treated with dignity and respect. The TPE is an

W.T. Choctaw, *Transforming the Patient Experience*,
DOI 10.1007/978-3-319-16928-6_1

action committee not a discussion committee, approximately half the members are management and half are physicians. As a result, we acknowledge the extraordinary work of many members of the TPE committee. We have learned that as we transform ourselves we transform our patient's experience.

Our TPE committee has evolved into our Patient Family Advisory Council (PFAC), further supporting and integrating the principle of patient centricity.

Chapter 2
The Power of Common Ground

The CEO and the Surgeon

In the fall of 2008 there was a buzz around Citrus Valley that the Board of Directors had hired a new CEO. Having been a member of the medical staff for over 25 years I was not terribly excited about this prospect. There was always excitement about new CEO's at the time but to me they were basically all alike. They would always appear professional usually nice and say the right things. They always talked about how important the doctors were and how determined they were to partner with the physicians. In my experience, however nothing ever really changed. The new CEO would usually last about 4–7 years then they would move on. Nevertheless, the hospital's Director of Strategic Planning was particularly enthusiastic about this new administrator, because she believed him to be physician oriented and I would like him.

Over the years, I have held a number of elected medical staff leadership positions at our hospital and had the opportunity to work closely with many of our previous hospital leaders. They were all intelligent people but I was never convinced they were genuinely interested in working with the physicians or making substantive changes. Nevertheless, some believed that this new CEO was what many of us physicians were waiting for and that he would work with physicians as equal partners. I had mentioned there always seems to be a disconnect between what was said and what was actually done. Sometime later, there was a meet and greet for the new CEO, I attended, more out of a sense of duty than anything else since I was the Chief of Surgery at the time. He was friendly and personable as I expected. A few weeks after the introductory reception, he sent a letter to all the attendees, offering to meet with any of us on an individual basis at any time and on any issue. After getting this general letter, I called the CEO's office and told him I would like to meet with him for 1 hour every other month for 6 months. He readily agreed. We began meeting as planned. I noticed however some things almost immediately that were somewhat surprising to me after the first couple of meetings. What I noticed was that he and I

W.T. Choctaw, *Transforming the Patient Experience*,
DOI 10.1007/978-3-319-16928-6_2

appeared to be surprisingly in agreement on most significant issues. The meetings were very relaxed and substantive. The next more important realization was that we were always philosophical in agreement. We have different styles but on substance, we were in complete agreement about important issues. Issues like patient centered quality care, patient's right, and staff and physician engagement. I began my primary practice here in the State of California. In California we have a long history of medical staff distrust of hospitals and predictable subsequent litigation. I generally viewed hospital CEOs and management executives as the Dark Vader of the healthcare universe where as we physicians were the Luke Skywalkers of the healthcare universe. Thus, this shared commonality of purpose and intent was very surprising to me. Nevertheless, we reached a level of mutuality. As a team of two, we had found common ground.

In January 2010, the new chief of staff asked me to chair a Physician Satisfaction Committee. We had never really had a very active Physician Satisfaction Committee. I told the new chief of staff that I would consider it. After consideration for a few days, I told him that I would do it, however, I wanted to set up my own particular guidelines for who I would invite and how I would proceed. He agreed. The first call I made to serve on the Physician Satisfaction Committee was the new CEO, Rob Curry. I explained to him the details of the committee and what it was designed to do. I told him I would like for him to be a member of the committee. He readily agreed. I then said to him that I did not want him to bring any additional staff or representatives of the management team. I wanted only him, in a room, with 15 physicians that I would choose to discuss various physician satisfaction issues. He also agreed. I then contacted the other members of the medical staff who represented a diverse spectrum of physicians, to meet with the CEO once a month to discuss physician concerns. We would meet regularly every month. At the first meeting, however, after much discussion about various issues from each physician, I noticed that Rob had a paperback book and that he was frequently flipping the pages. At the end of the meeting, he was given the opportunity to make comments and he did. When he finished, he said "I want to make sure that all of you read this book." He opined that many of the issues discussed in the meeting were already addressed in the book. At the conclusion of his comments, he remarkably, gave me his personal copy of the book and committed to purchase a copy for each of the 15 members of the committee. The book was entitled "Engaging Physicians" written by Dr. Stephen Beeson from Sharp Hospital in San Diego, California.

Dr. Beeson is a practicing family medicine physician with the Sharp-Stealy Medical Group. He is a member of the Studer Group. A nationally acclaimed leader committed to patient centered healthcare. Dr. Beeson's publication's intended purpose was to help hospitals and physicians:

- Create and boldly project a compelling organizational vision
- Assemble a high performance leadership structure, built to achieve outcomes based on a proven evidence-based model
- Select, develop, and activate physician champions to lead change

- Train and develop physicians using proven behaviors that dramatically improve clinical care and patient experience.
- Use performance feedback and data reporting to physicians to drive and improve quality and service outcomes
- Create, communicate, and implement physician behavioral standards consistent with an organizational vision
- Manage disruptive physicians in a proactive, fair, and consistent manner
- Recognize physicians in a way that generates physician organizational loyalty

After that initial meeting, I took the Dr. Beeson's book that Rob had given me and I read it completely the following weekend. It was amazing to me the information that had already been published in the literature regarding physician satisfaction issues and how to engage physicians. While reading Dr. Beeson's book, I would loudly exclaim words of joy and agreement. During this process of my weekend reading, my wife would frequently check on me to make sure I was not losing my sanity. Indeed. I had just finished a weekend of enlightenment! We used this book as if it were resource material for a postdoctoral class. Each physician member of the committee would read a chapter in the book and report to the committee at the next meeting. We would all discuss the chapter and analogize it with our own hospital.

We continued to meet monthly as the Physician Satisfaction Committee with Rob in attendance. We discussed various issues and toward the end of the first year, for the first time, we were able to get our own HCAHPS scores in committee. Subsequently Dr. Beeson has been invited to drive up from San Diego and speak at our hospital many times. On one occasion at our Strategic Planning Board of Director's Retreat, he was asked how long on average it took to engage physicians. He noted that they had been improving patient care and trying to improve their Hospital Consumer Assessment of Healthcare Providers and Systems (HCAHPS) scores at Sharp for a number of years. However, about 3 years into their efforts they realized that they had not included the physicians. He was asked how long it took to have physicians engaged and he said it took them approximately 5 years.

We are presently 3 years into our process to engage our physicians. Ironically, some of our major challenges are from the elected medical staff leadership. Some are totally invested in fighting the battles of the 1980s and are completely oblivious to the physician realities of twenty-first century healthcare. Nevertheless, the majority of our doctors on the medical staff are more interested in patient care and practice survival than hospital politics.

Chapter 3
Relentless Pursuit of "0" Harm

The Relentless Pursuit of "0"

There was a seismic shift in healthcare philosophy in 1998, when the Institute of Medicine (IOM) released its landmark study "to err is human". They noted that 48–98,000 patients die in hospitals yearly because of preventable mistakes. No other industry would accept this level of injury. For the first time, patient safety was elevated to the level of quality patient care. Significantly, this study shifted the healthcare debate from the vague grey area discussions of quality care for healthcare professionals, to the clear black and white area discussions of patient safety which any person or patient could understand. Under the most pedantic circumstances, any person knows that if they or their family member develops an injury, infection or preventable illness while in our hospital, we did not keep them safe.

The Joint Commission (TJC), the premier hospital regulatory organization in the country, codified this safety principle by making patient safety equal to quality care as a requirement for hospital certification. As leaders, managers and clinicians, we know TJC affirmation is not necessary. We long ago learned the golden rule of patient care: do no harm and treat patients the way we want to be treated. Our commitment exceeds the regulatory and rises to the level of the moral and the ethical. We honor this rule, by simply doing what is right for our patients and their families.

At CVHP, our transformation is vertical. Under the courageous leadership of Rob Curry, our CEO, and support from our Board of Directors, we have committed to become a High Reliability Organization (HRO). The fundamental principle of HRO's is "0" patient harm. We believe that "0" harm and quality patient care are fundamental rights all our patients have. We have added "safe" to our Mission Statement which now reads: To help people keep well in body, mind and spirit by providing quality healthcare services in a safe and compassionate environment. To reach this higher level of reliability in quality and safety, we have partnered with the Center for Transforming Healthcare (CTH), from the Joint Commission

W.T. Choctaw, *Transforming the Patient Experience*,
DOI 10.1007/978-3-319-16928-6_3

(TJC). They have contractually agreed to educate, train, and monitor our progress for 12 consecutive months. They have trained our senior leaders as a core team. The CTH helped us implement robust process improvement (RPI) including lean six sigma (LSS) methodology in 2014. RPI is about our people and our culture. We will trained at least 2 Black Belts and 20 Green Belts in-house. It has been said: "Give a man a fish he eats fish for a day, teach a man how to fish he eats fish for a lifetime."

During our first RPI year, TJC taught us how to fish. We learned that many of our quality and patient safety challenges are caused by ineffective, outdated and counterproductive processes.

We are determined to do better and reach high reliability. Our resolve is strong and our cause is just. Our patients deserve no less than "0" harm.

Robust Process Improvement

Our CVHP Transformation journey continues. We are committed to become a high reliability organization (HRO). As of June 2014, we have trained all our senior leaders, bi-weekly as a core team. The following activity has also occurred:

- One black Belt and 20 Green Belt candidates have been selected.
- Four physician champion leaders are among the lean six sigma candidates.
- Lean six sigma projects were selected using the criteria matrix.
- Lean six sigma Advisory Council was developed as an operational unit for the RPI/LSS Deployment leader.
- Lean Six Sigma Leadership Academy began training all middle level hospital employee leaders including hospital directors, managers and supervisors.

(See Chap. 6 for more on RPI process.)

Chapter 4
The Patient Experience

There are few things more terrifying than being a patient in a hospital. This imposed dependency is not only disorienting but extremely unsettling. Fear seizes the principal and his supportive family. The fear of surviving the episode is first followed closely by the fear of pain. Dr. Berwick, Founder of the Institution of Healthcare Improvement describes the patient's request as "cure me, don't hurt me, and be nice to me" as the frequent patient lament. Controlling pain is definitely within our skill set as healthcare providers. Nevertheless, we frequently fail miserably to adequately treat patient's pain. The patient perception of pain is so important that it has been added as the fifth vital sign by state legislators and is prominent in the 27 questions from the Hospital Consumer Assessment of Healthcare Providers and Systems (HCAHPS). Here, we concluded appropriate pain management was equal to quality patient care. We further decided as an organization that painful suffering would no longer be tolerated as a part of our patient's experience. At CVHP, we discovered proper pain management was not a new concept in our hospitals but the proper implementation of a system wide pain management program had never been effectively done. We created a single multiple disciplinary pain management protocol throughout our healthcare delivery system, supervised by a system wide pain management committee. Few elements impact the in-hospital patient experience more than pain management. As doctors, we need to set aside our anachronistic M.D. physician centered pain management approach.

The Beryl Institute defines the patient experience as "the sum of … all interactions, shaped by an organization's culture that influence patient perceptions across the continuum of care."

W.T. Choctaw, *Transforming the Patient Experience*,
DOI 10.1007/978-3-319-16928-6_4

Pain Protocol

The CVHP pain protocol has been activated at each of our three hospitals. The purpose of the protocol is to eliminate unnecessary pain and suffering among our patients. It is designed to cover all levels of pain including breakthrough pain. The pain protocol is also designed to eliminate unnecessary telephone calls to our physicians for pain medication (see Fig. 6.1). Pain management is an essential element in any patient and family's hospital experience. Various CVHP patient surveys continue to tell us we need to do a better job managing our patient's pain.

The pain protocol was initially a blue paper official order form, placed in each patient chart for verbal and written orders. It has subsequently been placed in our Electronic Health Record (EHR). The pain team including Rob and myself, continue to regularly make clinical rounds at each hospital to assure implementation and improvement. We can do better, we shall do better, and we must do better, because our patients deserve it.

Improving pain management is an essential element in transforming our patient's experience for better quality care. Quality pain control is one of those elements that transcend all specialties. We have a tremendous opportunity to improve our patient's pain experience as they journey through our facilities. Moreover, we began an ongoing system wide education program for all physicians, nurses, and staff about pain management at CVHP. Decreasing our patient's level of pain more effectively, will significantly improve our patient's care quality and satisfaction.

CVMC Adult Services

Acute Pain Management Orders (Outside of E.D.)

When ordering, physician must take into account other patient conditions that may influence use of drug or dosing of drug (age, obesity, sleep apnea, etc) and potential special monitoring that may be needed. Dose ranges given are approximate and may be higher based on patient weight and condition.

Pain Level 1-3:

- Tylenol 650 mg q6 h PRN mild pain. (May use with Ibuprofen if ordered.)
- If Tylenol ineffective within 1 h, give Norco (5/325) 1 tab PO × 1 dose. May repeat twice in a 24 h period.
- Ibuprofen 400 mg q6 h PRN mild pain. (May use with Tylenol if ordered.)
- Morphine____mg (0.5–2 mg) (0.013 mg/kg) IVP q2 h PRN **(If unable to take PO)**
- Toradol 30 mg IVP q6 h PRN. (Do not use for greater than 5 days) **(If unable to take PO)**

Dosing will be adjusted by pharmacy based on Medical Staff Protocol for age, weight, and renal function.
Caution in patients with GI ulcers, bleeding, antiplatelets or anticoagulants, and pts with CHF or cardiomyopathy).

Pain Level 4-6:

- Norco (5/325) **2** tab PO q6 h PRN (Do not give with Tylenol)
- ***If patient ≤55 years***: Morphine ___mg (1–3 mg) (0.03 mg/kg) IVP q2 h PRN **(If unable to take PO)**
- ***If patient >55 years***: Morphine____mg (0.5–2 mg) (0.013 mg/kg) IVP q2 h PRN **(If unable to take PO)**

Pain Level 7-10:

- ***If patient ≤55 years***: Morphine____mg (2–5 mg) (0.05 mg/kg) IVP q2 h PRN
- ***If patient >55 years***: Morphine ____mg (1–3 mg) (0.03 mg/kg) IVP q2 h PRN
- Tylenol 650 mg PO q6 h PRN ***in addition to Morphine***. (May give regardless of when narcotic was administered.)
- Tylenol 1 g IVPB q6 h PRN (max of 3 doses/24 h) ***in addition to Morphine***. **(If unable to take PO)** (May give regardless of when narcotic was administered.)
- Benadryl 25 mg IV × 1 dose with **first** dose of Morphine for ***any*** pain level.

Routine Ancillary Medications:

- Tylenol 650 mg q6 h PO. Add to narcotic regimen for Pain level 4–10. May administer at any time regardless of when last dose of narcotic given. **Do not use if Norco is administered more than twice a day.**
- Ibuprofen _____ mg (600–800 mg) q8 h PO routinely. May be used regardless of any administration of Tylenol or narcotics. **Do not use if Toradol being administered.**

For Breakthrough Pain:

- ***If patient ≤55 years***: Morphine____mg (1–3 mg) (0.03 mg/kg) IVP, 1 h after last dose of Morphine or Norco if pain >4 **(If needed more than twice in 24 h, call Physician)**
- ***If patient >55 years***: Morphine____mg (0.5–2 mg) (0.013 mg/kg) IVP, 1 h after last dose of Morphine or Norco if pain >4 **(If needed more than twice in 24 h, call Physician)**
- Benadryl 25 mg IV × 1 dose with **first** dose of Morphine
- Toradol 30 mg IVP q6 h PRN × 5 days **(Do NOT order if Toradol was ordered for Pain Level 1–3)**

Dosing will be adjusted by pharmacy based on Medical Staff Protocol for age, weight, and renal function.
Caution in patients with GI ulcers, bleeding, antiplatelets or anticoagulants, and pts with CHF or cardiomyopathy).

Other Medication:

- Benadryl 25 mg PO q6 h PRN for itching (caution: confusion in elderly)
- Benadryl 25 mg IV q6 h PRN for itching if PO route not available (caution: confusion in elderly)

- Hydroxyzine HCL 25 mg PO q6 h for itching
- Hydroxyzine HCL 25 mg IM q6 h for itching if PO route unavailable
- Zofran 4 mg IVP q6 h PRN for N/V
- Colace 100 mg PO BID—hold for loose stools
- Senna 2 tabs PO daily PRN constipation

Pain assessment: Pain must be assessed at least ONE HOUR after any pain med is given to determine if response has been adequate and if more meds are needed.

Narcan to reverse narcotic adverse events is available in all narcotic stock. Use as directed by nursing protocol or physician order.

Pain Bridge Protocol

Although our pain protocol was measuredly successful throughout our hospitals, we were still not meeting all our patient pain needs and reaching our goal to eliminate painful suffering. There were a large number of patients who were still suffering from pain because the physician forgot to write pain medicine orders or did not respond to nurse calls for additional pain medication for the patient as needed. Our pharmacy director suggested we develop a pain bridge. The pain bridge is in essence a pharmacy consult protocol. If, as an example, a surgeon operates on a patient and does not prescribe adequate pain medication, the nurse calls the M.D. for additional orders. If more than 30 min have passed and the physician has not answered, the nurse can place a pharmacy consult 24 h and 7 days a week using the pain bridge protocol policy. The pharmacist assesses the patient with the nurse and gives a one-time pain medication order, until the doctor calls. If more time passes and the doctor has not called, the nurse can repeat the consult as per the pain bridge protocol. Surprisingly, the use of the pain bridge protocol has soared at our hospitals. More than 100 of our patients have received better pain management directly because of the pain bridge protocol over a 6-month period. It suggested the pain management problem was even larger than we anticipated.

Bridging Pain Management Pharmacy Protocol

Purpose: To help patients ages 16 and above (exception: OB patients) alleviate severe pain in circumstances when they have either no orders for pain medication or the pain medication is not due to be given and the physician is unavailable for new orders.

Policy/Procedure:

1. If a patient reports severe pain (level of 7 or above) for a primary or secondary diagnosis and there is no pain medication ordered on the profile or the pain medication is not due to be given yet, the RN will contact the physician for additional orders for pain relief.
2. If the physician has not given any orders within 30 min and the patient remains in severe pain the RN will call the pharmacist for an order for a supplemental dose of an analgesic. RN will put in another call to the physician for additional orders.
3. The pharmacist will confirm with the RN the patients current pain level, when last analgesic was given and the effects of it and patients current weight. The patient will be assessed for any medications and conditions/co-morbidities that would contraindicate pain medications or alter dosing of pain medications (e.g. OSA, sedative hypnotic use, etc.)
4. The pharmacist will calculate and order one supplemental dose of analgesic using the following guidelines:Morphine 20–50 μg/kg IVP×1 (may give IM if no IV access) (Drug of choice)Hydromorphone 2–5 μg/kg IVP×1 (may give IM if no IV access) (If patient is intolerant to Morphine)Meperidine 25 mg IVP×1 (may give IM if no IV access) (to be used only if patient is truly allergic to Morphine)
5. RN to re-evaluate pain level within 60 min.
6. If patients pain level remains above 7 and there are no other pain medications available to be given and the physician has not yet given additional orders the RN may call the pharmacist for an additional dose of analgesic 1× only. (At least 30 min after the last dose.)
7. If the physician declines to order additional analgesics this protocol will not be initiated.
8. A Pharmacist will follow up with the RN/patient to assess the effects of the supplemental dose.

Chronic Pain Management Is a Palliative Care Journey

A few years ago, I operated on a patient with abdominal pain and a palpable abdominal mass. At the time of surgery, he was found to have a large carcinoma of the colon with advanced stage 4 metastasis. He had appropriate surgical resection and chemotherapy treatment. The following year, he had repeated hospital admissions related to his disease and chemotherapy treatment. Although my knowledge of advanced palliative care was limited, I asked him if he was willing to speak to a palliative care specialist to evaluate all his options. Initially he declined. However, months later, he and his wife both agreed. I asked Dr. Bruce Weimer (neurologist) to see him. The patient and his family were very pleased with the consultation. Dr. Weimer improved his chronic pain challenges and assisted with other end of life issues.

Although the above case deals with advanced palliative care and end of life issues, basic palliative care does not. Basic palliative care is merely symptomatic treatment irrespective of disease. For example, quality chronic pain management is basic palliative care. Palliative care is not hospice but the relief of symptomatic pain and suffering regardless of diagnosis. Many patients who frequent our facility have chronic pain conditions. They often are considered to be drug addicts because of their knowledge of pain medicine and frequent requests for medication. In general, some healthcare providers, doctors and nurses, treat these patients poorly because of societies' bias against perceived drug addiction. In reality, many of these patients are not addicts but have a chronic condition which accounts for their detailed knowledge of medications that help them. This perceived addiction bias allows many providers to justify allowing some patients to suffer.

An example of this misguided approach is demonstrated by the following hypothetical example: Nurse Nancy is a 42-year-old single parent who has two children. She is a medical surgery nurse who frequently works extra shifts to pay her bills and provide for her family. She has migraine headaches which she has had for 10 years. She has had a complete workup by a neurologist. At 1:00 am she gets a severe migraine headache causing her to go to the local emergency room (ER) close to her home. When she is finally seen after a prolonged wait in the waiting room, she tells the evaluating Registered Nurse that she is a nurse and that, she has been diagnosed with migraine headaches in the past by her neurologist. Hoping to expedite her care, she relates that when her migraines reach her present level of intensity, the medication that works is Dilaudid 2 mg IV. As soon as she mentions this narcotic with dosage, the evaluating nurse becomes more distant and appears to stop listening. She reassures nurse Nancy that she will be fine and the doctor will see her shortly. The nurse also tells her the doctor ordered some Toradol to decrease her pain. Somewhat upset, Nurse Nancy tells the ER nurse that Toradol does not work for her, only Dilaudid 2 mg! Nurse Nancy is trying to be helpful by impressing the ER team with her clinical knowledge. Nevertheless, the more she tries, the ER nurse sees her more as a desperate drug addict craving narcotic medication.

We are aggressively pursuing these areas in our hospitals with education and appropriate accountability tools.

Thank You to Our Patients

The essence of our transformation as a health care delivery system has been recognition of the importance of our patient's satisfaction. Nationally, patient satisfaction is now a major force in every part of healthcare. Gone are the days of doctor and nurse paternalism. The days when patients had minimal input into the process or choice over their medical care or the care that their families might receive. Patient satisfaction scores across the country now specifically define quality care from the patient's perspective. Many national consulting firms are giving conferences, seminars, webinars, etc., to advise hospitals, doctors and nurses about how to improve their patient satisfaction scores (HCAPHS). Many books and articles have been written on the same subject. I think the approach should be very basic. I believe an important place to start to improve patient satisfaction and quality care is for doctors to get in the habit of saying thank you more often. The words are basic but powerful. We should say thank you to our office staff, hospital employees, nurses, and especially our patients. As physicians, we are given a tremendous amount of respect from our healthcare team and patients. We should always reciprocate with Thank You. Sometimes a few respectful words from the doctor is all the patient wants in return.

Chapter 5
Physician Champions

Accountability

Having been in practice for over 30 years, I have seen many changes in the healthcare industry landscape, especially from the perspective of the practicing physician. Many of my surgical and medical colleagues frequently bemoan the state of US healthcare; they talk about the good old days of the past. As physicians, we tend to blame everyone else (Obama, hospital administrators, politicians, patients, etc.) for the chaotic state of our country's healthcare but we never appear to take collective responsibility ourselves. The reality is we physicians abdicated our leadership role in national healthcare by opining we would just take care of patients and not get involved with politics. We physicians, incorrectly, assumed we were special and would never be significantly affected by what was and is happening on the national stage. Nevertheless, national health alignment was occurring between patients/families, political leaders, payers, and technology. Had we physicians looked outside our "Hippocratic castles," we would have seen much of this coming. Fundamental, to much of the healthcare change is the basic concept of patient centered care. Care is centered on the needs and concerns of the patient not the needs and concerns of the doctor. This simple concept is frequently lost in physician group discussions.

Unfortunately, now as we continue to helplessly complain about national health affairs, we codify our irrelevance at the medical staff leadership level by clinging to anachronistic ideas. Ideas such as; Healthcare reform will go away, it's about the doctor and not the patient. If we are to collectively have a more prominent leadership role, we must hold ourselves more accountable.

W.T. Choctaw, *Transforming the Patient Experience: A New Paradigm for Hospital and Physician Leadership*, DOI 10.1007/978-3-319-16928-6_5

A key element of accountability is good data. The most influential data in healthcare is patient satisfaction data call HCAHPS. It codified the concept of patient centered care because the Center for Medicare/Medicaid Service began to tie the HCAHPS score to reimbursement for hospitals and physicians. I had sat in many meetings at CVHP listening to issues about the variation of our hospitals HCAHPS scores. As a practicing physician my interest in this survey was distant, then I got an idea that what we should do at CVHP is to send physicians their individual scores to their offices by mail. I presented the idea to Rob and he thought it was great. I then began to investigate how to actually do that with the hospital data. I was told repeatedly that it could not be reasonably done. Nevertheless, I persisted. One of my major lessons learned from Rob is to be "relentless." I finally found an assistant who gave me hope when she said "Dr. Choctaw, I don't know how to do it but I can figure it out." I like people who are willing to figure things out. I call these type of employees, Superstars. Her name is Denise Ronquillo. A few years later I hired her to be my Corporate Director of Process Excellence (see Chap 8).

The physician reaction to receiving their own scores were predictably mixed. The scores ranged from 1 to 99. The highest score is the best. The physicians with high scores were happy, those with low scores were deeply offended. The low HCAHPS physicians would yell at me over the phone or complain to me face to face in the Doctors' lounge. They would tell me how they are good doctors, how their patients love them, some would mention how much money they donate to the hospital. I would respectfully respond that I know they are good doctors and their patients love them. I would further tell them that all the HCAHPS survey does is measure the patient's perception of how well the doctor communicates with their patient. The survey asks three basic questions about the physician:

- How often did your doctor treat you with courtesy and respect
- How often did your doctor listen to you
- How often did your doctor explain in ways you understand

The patients are asked to respond: Never, Sometimes, Usually, or Always. The Always score is the only choice recorded.

However, the high HCAHPS physicians in the 99 percentile were my new best friends. They would smile and wave at me in the hospital parking lot. Importantly, our goal was achieved. The goal was to educate physicians about patient satisfaction and the patient's perception of quality regarding physician communication. The HCAHPS survey was at the core of our CVHP Physician Coaches Team activity. Much of our coaching is about helping doctors communicate better with their patients to improve safety and the quality of care. Some techniques we coach are: having doctors sit when they talk to patients, introduce themselves, and be respectful to patients and their families. We also coach physicians in the art of giving patients permission to ask questions by saying "do you have any questions, I have the time." Our physician Coaching Program is not peer review. We coach physicians, one on one, to prevent peer review. The implementation of the HCAHPS patient satisfaction survey is exemplary of how we physicians are being held accountable like never before.

Physicians Must Lead

There is strong leadership from the federal government to get something done in the area of health care reform. In the latest issue of the National Journal, Ronald Brownstein examines the steps the Obama Administration is taking to engage stakeholder groups on key legislative issues and how President Obama's "inclusive nature" may yield dividends for health care reform.

Recently, a group of national stakeholders in health care reform met with President Obama and pledged to decrease health care costs by more than 2 trillion dollars over the next 10 years. A savings of $2,500 for each American family would result. The group plans to reach this goal by focusing on five main areas:

1. Improving care after hospitalizations and reducing hospital readmission rates
2. Reducing Medicare overpayments to private insurers through competitive payments
3. Reducing drug prices
4. Improving Medicare and Medicaid payment accuracy
5. Expanding the Hospital Quality Improvement Program

Healthcare cost reduction will occur, if the process has broader physician leadership. The process must remain patient friendly and protective. No longer should the MD and MBA be "mutually exclusive." Doctors are potentially the strongest patient advocates because of the doctor-patient relationship and their relative independence in providing care.

It is imperative that physicians regain some influence if not full control of the dictionary. We can start to do this by doing some of the following:

- Become more knowledgeable about healthcare issues by watching more CSPAN and less CNN and FOX News.
- Actively participating in medical staff leadership positions in our hospitals by becoming; chief of staff, chief of medicine, etc.
- Redefine the words in healthcare legislation by running for political office instead of retiring at age 60.

And most importantly, we physicians have a moral, ethical, and legal imperative to commit to health care reform and patient centered care quickly.

Physician Coaches

Nationally, hospitals are all evaluating ways to partner with the active doctors on their medical staff. However, true partnership will not occur without true physician philosophical alignment. Doctors must be aligned with the mission, visions, and values of the organization. At CVHP, under the leadership of Rob Curry, CEO, and collaboration of the executive management team and Board of Directors, we have developed a process to provide patient-centered quality care with medical staff leaders. Our process is similar to that described by Dr. Stephen Beeson in his book "Engaging Physicians." There are three basic categories of physician leaders in a healthcare organization. They are the elected leaders, the informal leaders, and the physician champion leaders. Our CVHP coaches are physician champion leaders. Physician champions are active staff physicians specifically trained to assist with the implementation of quality, safety, and service initiatives. At CVHP, we have selected a highly skilled team to be physician coaches. Our coaches have the following requisite qualities:

- They are driven by a value system that is always patient centered. They believe quality care is a fundamental patient right.
- They are progressive thinkers who understand the modern healthcare delivery system.
- They possess the ability to communicate CVHP's pillar based quality strategy.
- They have the ability to create consensus.
- They possess the ability to stand when challenged.
- They promote the ideals of system based care.
- They are driven by the passions to transform the patient experience.

Our coaches represent a variety of specialties and practice at all three of our hospitals. They all completed a mandatory Physician Leadership Academy program and continue to receive ongoing training in a variety of areas such as Press Ganey etc. Some of the goals of the peer to peer coaching team are:

- Improve patient satisfaction
- Improve physician satisfaction
- Improve Physician/nurse/administration collaboration
- Improve implementation and compliance with evidence based clinical protocols
- Improve physician accountability

Presently, coaching activity has involved physician to patient communication issues, patient complaints and new physicians to the CVHP medical staff. To date over 100 physicians have been coached by the team. Our purpose is to transform our patient experience by respectfully assisting our physicians. Our coaches must have certain core characteristics.

Physician Leadership Development

Today's healthcare delivery systems require strong physician partners to survive. Organizations are undergoing transformation to meet this need. An essential element of this transformation is physician alignment. The alignment necessitates a solid structured physician development process. The intent is to provide a continuous ongoing education process for our physicians while implementing clinical integration.

Level I

- Peer to Peer Relationship
- Reorientation lectures
- Articles, webinars
- Class Activity Compassion Teamwork (ACT)
- All MD contracts include basic information

Level II

- Level I and
- Seminars, Conferences, Books
- Press Ganey Account Data to monitor physician satisfaction score
- Teaching, Presentations
- Peer to Peer Coaching
- Coach Academy Classes

The Physician Metrics Plan

Goal: To Transform the Patient's Experience at CVHP

Issue: Transforming Physicians is an essential element to transform the patient's experience at CVHP. Physician metrics is an indispensable tool to help transform doctors.

Step 1: Share all quality performance data with physicians personally.

- HCAPHS
- Core Measures
- Crimson Data

Step 2: Give physician appropriate tools to understand and use data.

- Publications—Fax-Facts, MDialogue, Physician-2-Physician Newsletter, TPE Report, etc.

(continued)

- Physician Satisfaction Committee information

Step 3: Develop team of Physician Coaches
Timeline

- September—TPE committee adopts and fine tunes plan
- October—HCAPHS scores sent to all clinical departments, develop reporting infrastructure, recruit MD Coaches
- November—formally report on physician metrics plan to both Medical Executive Committee and management team

Physician Leadership Coaches Retreat

Objectives

- Understand the role of good communication in quality patient care
- Apply new approaches to improve communication with patients
- Understand the impact of healthcare reform in CVHP and physicians
- Identify methods to transform the patient experience as a member of CVHP
- Mitigate medical legal problems from poor doctor patient communication

"Curry" Rounds

Rob Curry, CEO, is now making clinical patient experience rounds weekly. A historic occurrence for CVHP. He and I make the clinical rounds together. We sit with employees on rounds, we each take notes and then follow up on requests. Many topics are discussed including pain management, doctor/nurse/patient communication, nurse staffing, etc. The staff is excited and engaged. The rounds occur at all three hospitals.

Physician High Performer Characteristics

- Models CVHP Mission, Vision, and Values
- Supports Patient's Fundamental Right to Quality Care
- Patient Centered
- Trained CVHP Leadership Academy
- Collaborative
- Professional
- High HCAHPS Scores
- High Core Measure Scores
- CPOE/EHR User

Physician High Performer Development Program
Physicians are a Requirement to Transform the Patient's experience (Why)
Identify and Develop Physician High Performers (What)
Process (How)

1. Senior Rounding
   - Chief Transformation Officer
   - Chief Executive Officer
2. Education
   - Books—Engaging Physicians, HCAHPS, Hardwiring for Excellence, etc.
   - Conferences—Coaches Leadership Seminar, etc.
   - Webinars—Studer on physicians, etc.
3. Committee Team Participation
   - Transforming the Patient Experience Team
   - Physician Satisfaction Committee
   - Coaching Team
4. Physician Metrics—Physician Scorecard
   - HCAHPS
   - Core Measures
5. Lean Six Sigma Training

To comply with all state and federal regulations, it is important to have physician agreements in writing and reviewed by hospital legal counsel. The following is a sample written contract that codified the original agreement between physician coaches and hospital, with a sample letter of engagement.

(Sample Physician Contract)

PHYSICIAN COACHING SERVICES AGREEMENT

This PHYSICIAN COACHING SERVICES AGREEMENT ("**Agreement**"), dated as of the 1st day of _______ (the "**Effective date**"), is made by and between CITRUS VALLEY HEALTH PARTNERS, INC., a California non-profit corporation ("**CVHP**") and ______________________________________, M.D., an individual ("**Physician**"). CVHP and Physician are referred to herein individually as a "**party**" and, collectively, the "**parties**".

RECITALS

A. CVHP owns and operated three hospital campuses (collectively, the "**Hospitals**") and a hospice (the "**Hospice**" and, collectively with the Hospitals, the "**Facilities**").
B. Physician is licensed to practice medicine in California.

C. Physician champions are essential to coach medical staff members at the Facilities in helping them deliver quality care that is perceived to be thoughtful and compassionate.
D. All CVHP personnel, whether employees or physicians, play a key role in delivering quality care to patients.
E. A consistent standard of professionalism is expected to develop the CVHP brand that reflects quality, responsiveness, and value. The goal of this Agreement is to appropriately compensate physician coaches for their work and results in helping CVHP develop and maintain this consistent standard of professionalism across all physicians who work with CVHP and/or at the Facilities.
F. CVHP requires the services of Physician to provide certain physician coaching services to certain physicians who practice at the Facilities, as further described in this Agreement (collectively, the "**Services**").
G. CVHP and Physician desire to enter into this Agreement in order to provide a full statement of their respective rights and responsibilities in connection with the provision of the Services during the term of this Agreement and any extensions thereof.

NOW, THEREFORE, for good and valuable consideration, the receipt and sufficiency of which are hereby acknowledged, the parties to this Agreement agree as follows.

AGREEMENT
ARTICLE I
PHYSICIAN'S RESPONSIBILITIES

1.1 **Provision of the Services.** Physician shall provide or arrange for the Services set forth on Exhibit 1.1. Physician shall: (a) personally perform Services at the Facilities in which CVHP and Physician mutually agree; (b) perform all duties in accordance with the rules and policies, instructions, and protocols instituted from time to time by CVHP; (c) attend such training sessions as CVHP provides and/or requests in connection with the Services; (d) provide such oral and written reports as CVHP from time to time requires; and (e) perform to the full and complete satisfaction of CVHP.
1.2 **Scope of Services.** The Services rendered by Physician shall be (i) within the scope of Physician's licensure, qualifications and expertise; (ii) within the scope of Physician's clinical privileges at the Facilities if and as applicable; and (iii) consistent with accepted community standards of practice.
1.3 **Location and Schedule of Services.** Physician shall provide Services at such times and locations as Physician and CVHP may mutually agree from time to time.
1.4 **Physician Qualifications.** Physician represents and warrants that as of the Effective Date and throughout the term of this Agreement, Physician: (a) holds an unrestricted license to practice medicine in California from the Medical Board of California (b) holds an unrestricted federal Drug enforcement Agency ("**DEA**") number; (c) is not charged with, and has never been convicted of, a

felony, a misdemeanor involving moral turpitude, fraud, dishonesty, or controlled substances, or any healthcare-related crime, (d) is in good standing with, and has not been suspended, excluded, or debarred from, or otherwise rendered ineligible to participate in, in the Medicare and Medi-Cal Programs, and any other federally-funded health care program; (e) maintains professional liability insurance at least in the amounts set forth in this Agreement; (f) has not had any adverse peer review activity taken against Physician in the past 24 months; (g) has had no patient complaints in past 24 months that were upheld by peer review; (h) has had no behavioral concerns that necessitated action by a peer review committee or any health facility department.

1.5 **Notification of Certain Events.** Physician shall notify CVHP in writing within 3 business days following Physician's knowledge of the occurrence of any one or more of the following events: (a) Physician's medical staff membership or clinical privileges at any health facility are recommended for disciplinary action or are denied, suspended, restricted, revoked or voluntarily relinquished, regardless of the availability of civil or administrative hearing rights or judicial review with respect thereto; (b) Physician becomes the subject of any suit, action or other legal proceeding arising out of Physician's professional services; (c) Physician is required to pay damages or any other amount in any malpractice action by way of judgment or settlement; (d) Physician becomes the subject of any disciplinary proceeding or action before any state's medical board or similar agency responsible for professional standards or behavior; (e) Physician becomes incapacitated or disabled from performing the Services, or voluntarily or involuntarily retires from the practice of medicine (f) Physician is charged with, convicted of, or pleads nolo contendere to a felony criminal offense; (g) any act of nature or any other event occurs which Physician knows or reasonably should know has a material adverse effect on Physician's ability to provide the Services; (h) Physician is debarred, suspended or otherwise ineligible to participate in any federal or state health care program; or (i) Physician charges Specialty.

1.6 **Time Records.** Physician shall record promptly and maintain all information pertaining to Physician's performance of Services under this Agreement. Before the 15th day of the month following the month in which the Services were provided during the term of this Agreement, Physician shall submit to CVHP's Chief financial Officer or designee complete and accurate time records and certification of the time records substantially in the form attached hereto as Exhibit 1.3, and shall contain the information requested by CVHP. If complete and accurate time records and the corresponding certification are not received within 90 days following the end of the calendar month in which the Services were rendered. CVHP may deny payment to Physician. Notwithstanding the preceding provisions of this Section 1.6, to the extent CVHP maintains attendance records for any meetings, in-services, or other Services (as such services are defined in Exhibit 1.1), such attendance records shall constitute adequate documentation of Physician's performance of the Services if such records include the date, time, duration, specific nature of the Services provided, and note the name of Physician as being in attendance.

1.7 **CVHP Policies and Procedures.** Physician shall comply with all policies, procedures and protocols of CVHP, as adopted and/or amended by CVHP from time to time. CVHP may revise, supplement or terminate any policy, practice or procedure at any time in CVHP's sole discretion.

1.8 **Continuing Education and Professional Meetings.** Physician shall maintain Physician's professional competence and skills commensurate with the medical standards of the community and as required by law by attending and participating in approved continuing education courses.

1.9 **Regulatory Compliance.** Physician shall comply with all applicable provisions of state and federal law which prohibit discrimination in the provision of Services to applicable physicians on the basis of race, color, national origin, ancestry, religion, sex, marital status, sexual orientation age, or any other category protected by law. Physician shall render Services for all physicians designated by CVHP in the same manner and in accordance with the same standards and within the same time availability as Services are rendered to physicians who do not practice at the Facilities. Physician shall provide CVHP with such records and such other information as may be required by law or regulation relating to Services provided by Physician.

ARTICLE II
CVHP'S RESPONSIBILITIES

2.1 **Premises.** CVHP shall furnish throughout the term hereof such space as CVHP deems necessary for the proper and efficient provision of the Services. Notwithstanding anything herein to the contrary, CVHP may, from time to time, and at its discretion, charge, decrease, alter or replace said space.

2.2 **Personnel.** CVHP shall employ sufficient personnel required for the proper provision of the Services.

2.3 **Equipment.** CVHP shall provide, at its sole expense, all equipment it deems necessary for the efficient and safe provision of the Services. All such equipment shall at all times remain the property of CVHP. CVHP shall, at its sole cost and expense, maintain equipment and shall, within a reasonable time, replace any portion thereof which becomes worn out or obsolete with equipment similar or better in character and utility to that being replaced.

ARTICLE III
COMPENSATION AND BILLING

3.1 **Compensation.** As compensation to Physician for providing the Services. CVHP shall pay Physician pursuant to the terms set forth on <u>Exhibit 2.1.</u>

3.2 **Payment; Documentation Required.** Payment of compensation due to Physician under <u>Section 3.1</u> is expressly conditioned upon Physician complying with the documentation requirements set forth in <u>Section 1.6.</u> CVHP shall have no obligation to compensate Physician for any Services unless and until CVHP has received necessary and appropriate documentation within the timeframes set forth in <u>Section 1.6.</u> Subject to the preceding provisions, CVHP shall pay Physician the invoiced amount before the 15th day of the month following the month in which CVHP receives the invoice, provided that CVHP shall retain the right to audit and recalculate invoices at any time during the term of this Agreement and for a period of 7 years thereafter.

3.3 **Exclusive Source of Compensation for Services**. The compensation provided under this Agreement shall be the exclusive source of compensation to Physician for rendering the Services. Physician shall not bill, or cause to be billed, patients or any third-party payors (including, without limitation, the Medicare or Medicaid programs) for the Services. Physician shall indemnify, defend and hold harmless CVHP from and against any liability which CVHP may incur, including but not limited to attorneys' fees, arising or resulting from or incurred due to the billing of patients or third-party payors by Physician or any agent or employee of Physician.

3.4 **Fair Value Warranty.** Each party represents and warrants on behalf of itself, that the aggregate benefit given or received under this Agreement has been determined in advance through a process of arms-length negotiations that were intended to achieve an exchange of goods and/or services consistent with fair market value under the circumstances, and that any benefit given or received under this Agreement is not intended to induce, does not require, and is not contingent upon, the admission, recommendation or referral of any customer, directly or indirectly, and further, is not determined in any manner that takes into account the value of business generated between the parties.

ARTICLE V
TERM AND TERMINATION

5.1 **Term.** The initial term of this Agreement shall begin on the Effective Date and shall continue for a period of 1 year ("**Initial term**"), and thereafter this Agreement shall automatically renew for additional successive 1 year terms (each a "**Renewal Term**"), unless this Agreement is earlier terminated as provided herein. References herein to the "term" of this Agreement mean the Initial term and any renewal Term, as applicable. CVHP is not, by entering into this Agreement, promising Physician any minimum amount of work. CVHP shall have no obligation to provide Physician with any set number of days or work during any period and it is further understood that Physician will be scheduled to provide the Services solely on an "as needed basis" as requested by CVHP.

5.2 **Termination.** Notwithstanding any other provision in this agreement, this Agreement may be terminated upon the occurrence of any of the following:

(a) Termination for Breach. Either party may terminate this Agreement on 30 days' written notice to the other party if the party to whom such notice is given is in material breach of this Agreement. The party claiming the right to terminate hereunder shall set forth in the notice of intended termination the facts underlying its claim that the other party is in breach of this Agreement. Remedy of such breach within such 30 day notice period shall revive the Agreement in effect for the remaining term.

(b) Termination for Cause. If the overall CVHP HCAHPS score for physician communication fails to reach the 51st percentile by the December ____ reporting period, CVHP has the right to terminate this agreement with 30 days' written notice.
(c) Immediate Termination by CVHP. CVHP may, but shall not be obligated to, terminate this Agreement immediately by written notice to Physician upon the occurrence of any of the following events:

 (i) the failure of Physician to meet any of the qualifications set forth in Section 1.4;
 (ii) conduct by Physician which, in the reasonable discretion of CVHP, is deemed to be jeopardizing the health, safety, or well-being of any patient or the business of CVHP, including without limitation, acts of harassment against CVHP's staff or any Facility's staff or patients, or unlawful or unethical conduct; or
 (iii) Physician is charged with or convicted of any felony, any misdemeanor involving fraud, dishonesty, controlled substances, or moral turpitude, or any healthcare-related crime or misdemeanor.

Notwithstanding the preceding provisions of this Section 5.2(c)(i), Section 5.2(c)(iii), CVHP shall provide Physician with 5 business days' prior written notice of CVHP's intent to terminate under this Section, which notice shall set forth the basis for CVJP's intent to terminate. To the extent Physician cures, to CVHP's satisfaction, the basis for CVHP's intent to terminate within such 5 day period, such cure shall revive the Agreement in effect for the remaining term.

(a) Termination for Breach. Either party may terminate this Agreement on 30 days' written notice to the other party if the party to whom such notice is given is in material breach of this Agreement. The party claiming the right to terminate hereunder shall set forth in the notice of intended termination the facts underlying its claim that the other party is in breach of this Agreement. Reedy of such breach within such 30 day notice period shall revive the Agreement in effect for the remaining term.
(b) Termination for Cause. If the overall CVHP HCAHPS score for physician communication fails to reach the 51st percentile by the December ____ reporting period, CVHP has the right to terminate this agreement with 30 days' written notice.
(c) Immediate Termination by CVHP. CVHP may, but shall not be obligated to, terminate this Agreement immediately by written notice to Physician upon the occurrence of any of the following events;

 (i) The failure of Physician to meet any of the qualifications set forth in Section 1.4;
 (ii) Conduct by Physician which, in the reasonable discretion of CVHP, is deemed to be jeopardizing the health, safety, or wellbeing of any patient or the business of CVHP, including without limitation, acts of harassment against CVHP's staff or any Facility's staff or patients, or unlawful or unethical conduct; or

(iii) Physician is charged with or convicted of any felony, any misdemeanor involving fraud, dishonesty, controlled substances, or moral turpitude, or any healthcare-related crime of misdemeanor.

Notwithstanding the preceding provisions of this Section 5.2(c) prior to exercising its termination rights under Section 5.2(c)(i), Section 5.2(c)(ii), Section 5.2(c)(iii), CVHP shall provide Physician with 5 business days' prior written notice of CVHP's intent to terminate under this Section, which notice shall set forth the basis for CVHP's intent to terminate. To the extent Physician cures, to CVHP's satisfaction, the basis for CVHP's intent to terminate within such 5 day period, such cure shall revive the Agreement in effect for the remaining term.

(a) Termination Without Cause. Either party may terminate this Agreement for any reason or no reason on 60 days' prior written notice to the other party.
(b) Termination upon Legal Event. Notwithstanding any other provision of this Agreement, if the governmental agencies that administer the Medicare, Medicaid, or other federally funded programs (or their representatives or agents), or any other federal, state or local governmental or nongovernmental agency, or any court of administrative tribunal passes, issues or promulgates any law, rule, regulation, standard, interpretation, order, decision or judgment, including but hot limited to those relating to any regulations pursuant to state or federal anti-kickback or physician self-referral statutes (collectively or individually, "**Legal Event**"), which, in the good faith judgment of one party (the "**Noticing Party**"), materially and adversely affects either party's licensure, accreditation, certification, tax-exempt status, or ability to refer, to accept any referral, to bill, to claim, to present a bill or claim, or to receive payment of reimbursement from any federal, state or local governmental or nongovernmental payor, or to obtain tax-exempt financing, or which subjects the Noticing Party to a risk of prosecution of civil monetary penalty, or if in the good faith opinion of counsel to either party any term or provision

Of this Agreement could trigger a Legal Event, then the Noticing Party may give the other party notice of intent to amend or terminate this Agreement. If such notice occurs, the parties shall have 30 days from the giving of such notice ("**Renegotiation Period**") within which to attempt to amend this Agreement. If this Agreement is not so amended within the renegotiation Period, this Agreement shall terminate as of midnight on the 30th day after said notice was given. Except as otherwise required by applicable law, any amounts owing to either party hereunder shall be paid, on a pro rata basis, up to the date of such termination, and any obligation hereunder that is to continue beyond expiration or termination shall so continue pursuant to its terms.

5.3 **Effects of Expiration or Termination.** Upon expiration or termination of this Agreement neither party shall have any further obligation hereunder except for obligations arising prior to the date of termination and obligations, promises, or covenants contained herein which expressly extend beyond the term of this Agreement.

ARTICLE VI: INDEMNIFICATION

6.1 **Indemnification.** To the extent permitted by laws, each party shall indemnify, defend and hold harmless the other party and its agents, employees, contractors, officers and directors against: (i) any and all liability arising out of such party's failure to comply with the terms of this Agreement, and any injury, loss, claims, or damages arising from the negligent operations, acts, or omissions of such party or its employees relating to or arising out of this Agreement; and (ii) any and all costs and expenses, including reasonable legal expenses incurred by or on behalf of such party in connection with the defense of such claims. Each party shall cooperate with the other in the defense of any claim, demand or other matter and make available all information and assistance that the other party may reasonably request. The indemnification obligations under this Section shall only apply if and to the extent that such indemnified acts or omissions are not completely covered by insurance.

6.2 **Cooperation Between the Parties.**

(a) During the term of this Agreement and for a period hereafter, certain risk management issues, legal issues, claims or actions may arise that involve or could potentially involve the parties and their respective employees and agents. The parties recognize the importance of cooperating with each other in good faith when such issues, claims or actions arise, to the extent such cooperation does not violate any applicable laws, cause the breach of any duties created by any policies of insurance or programs of self-insurance, or otherwise compromise the confidentiality of communications or information regarding the issues, claims or actions, as such, the parties shall cooperate in good faith, using their best efforts, to address such risk management and claims handling issues in a manner that strongly encourages full cooperation between the parties.

(b) If a controversy, dispute, claim, action or lawsuit (each, and "**Action**") arises with a third party wherein both the parties are included as defendants, each party shall promptly disclose to the other party in writing the existence and continuing status of the Action and any negotiations relating thereto. Each party shall make every reasonable attempt to include the other party in any settlement offer or negotiations. In the event the other party is not included in the settlement, the settling party shall immediately disclose to the other party in writing the acceptance of any settlement and terms relating thereto.

ARTICLE VII
CONFIDENTIALITY

7.1 **Business Records.** Any and all business, financial, quality assurance, peer review, or other records pertaining to CVHP and its activities (collectively "**CVHP Records**") are and shall remain exclusively the property of CVHP. Physicians shall not have or acquire any interest or right in or to any CVHP Records whatsoever. No later than 3 days after the effective date of expiration or termination of this Agreement, Physician shall turn over to CVHP all correspondence, papers, patient date lists, writings and other CVHP records in Physician's possession or control pertaining to the finances, patients, practice or other activities of CVJP or which Physician received incident thereto or in connection with the performance of Physician's duties, unless physician in another capacity is entitled to retain any of such items.

7.2 **Confidentiality.** Physician shall keep confidential and shall not, either directly or indirectly, divulge, disclose or communicate to any person, firm, or entity, any proprietary information of CVHP, including without limitation, any list of CVHP's patients or of its professional plans, methods, strategies or arrangements of CVHP, or the terms of this agreement (collectively, "**Confidential Information**"), except as required by law, as expressly provided in this Agreement, or with the express advance written authorization by CVHP. Notwithstanding the foregoing, Physician may disclose Confidential Information to Physician's attorneys, accountants, or business advisers ("**Advisers**") on a need to now basis. Physician represents and warrants that: (i) any Advisers will comply with the confidentiality provision, (ii) physician will obtain from advisers all agreements or assurances required under HIPAA or other federal and state laws governing the confidentiality of health information; and (iii) no adviser will further disclose any Confidential Information except as required by laws.

7.3 **Non-Solicitation.** During and after termination of this Agreement, Physician shall not, directly or indirectly, for any reason, use any Confidential Information for any purpose competitive with CVHP or otherwise inconsistent with the purposes of this Agreement, including the solicitation of business from any third-party payor, employer group, member, enrollee or patient of any third-party payor, or the solicitation of any employee or contractor of CVHP to terminate such person's employment or contract with CVHP. In the event of a breach or threatened breach by physician of the provisions of this Section, CVHP shall be entitled to an injunction restraining Physician from disclosing, in whole or in part, the Confidential Information, or from otherwise violating this section. Nothing in this agreement shall be construed so as to prevent CVHP from pursuing any other remedies available to either of them for any disclosure or solicitation in violation of this Section, including the recovery of damages from Physician.

ARTICLE VIII
DISPUTE RESOLUTION

8.1 **In General.** All controversies, claims, disputes and counterclaims arising out of, relating to or in connection with this Agreement, whether based on statute, tort, contract, common law or otherwise ("**Dispute**"), shall be resolved by binding arbitration as set forth in this Section. Any party to this Agreement may commence binding arbitration as described herein to resolve a Dispute.

8.2 **Rules.** Arbitration of the dispute shall be resolved by binding arbitration pursuant to the Judicial Arbitration and Mediation Service ("**JAMS**") then-current Streamlined Arbitration Rules and Procedures, a copy of which is available at http;://www.jamsadr.com/rules-streamlined-arbitration/ (the "**Rules**").

8.3 **Selection of Arbitrator Location of Arbitration** The arbitration shall be conducted before a single arbitrator who shall be a retired judicial officer, as mutually agreed by the parties. If the parties cannot agree on a single arbitrator, the arbitrator shall be selected pursuant to the rules. The arbitration shall be held at JAMS's Los Angeles office or at any other location the parties mutually agree.

8.4 **Governing Law; Discovery; Award.** The laws of the State of California shall govern the substantive rights of the parties in the arbitration proceeding. By agreeing to arbitration, the parties are waiving all rights to seek remedies in court. The arbitrator shall have jurisdiction over the Dispute, and the decision of the arbitrator shall be final and binding upon the parties. Depositions may be taken and discovery may be conducted in the manner to give each party a reasonable opportunity to conduct discovery, as designated by the arbitrator with good cause shown by the parties. The arbitrator's award shall include the arbitrator's written reasoned opinion, and the arbitrator shall not have the power to commit errors of law or legal reasoning.

8.5 **Appeal of Award.** At the request of either party within 14 calendar days after issuance of the award, the award shall be subject to affirmation, reversal or modification, following review of the record and arguments of the parties by a single second arbitrator who shall, as far as practicable, proceed in accordance with the law and procedures applicable to appellate review by the California Court of Appeal of a civil judgment following a court trial. Any such appeal shall be conducted pursuant to the then-current JAMS Optional Arbitration Appeal Procedure, a copy of which is available on the HAMS website at http://www.jamsadr.com/rules-optional-appeal-procedure/.

8.6 **Fees and Costs Entry of Judgment.** In any arbitration held pursuant to this Agreement, all fees and costs of arbitration, including the arbitrator's fee, shall be allocated in accordance with the Rules, except that in no case shall Physician's share of such fees and costs exceed the then-current total filing fee and costs in any court in which Physician could have filed suit. The arbitrator may award reasonable attorneys' fees to the prevailing party to the extent such award is not inconsistent with statutory or case law. Judgment upon the arbitration award may be entered in any court having jurisdiction, or application may be made by either party to such court for a judicial acceptance of the award and an order of enforcement, as applicable.

8.7 **Provisional Remedies.** This Section shall not limit the right of any party under California Code of Civil Procedure Section 1281.8 to obtain or oppose provisional or ancillary remedies, including, without limitation, temporary restraining orders, injunctive relief, and such other provisional relief as a court of competent jurisdiction may deem appropriate (collectively, "**Provisional Remedies**"), before the commencement of arbitration proceedings under this Agreement. After the arbitration proceedings have commenced or while such proceedings are pending, the arbitrator shall have the power to grant Provisional

Remedies as the arbitrator may deem appropriate and may modify any previously granted Provisional Remedies.

8.8 **Negotiation or Mediation.** The parties may, by mutual written agreement, stay the commencement of the arbitration procedure from time to time to allow for any form of negotiation or mediation of the Dispute.

8.9 **Availability of Arbitration Rules and Procedures.** Physician has had the opportunity to review the Rules, local office locations, and appeal procedure referenced in this Section. Physician may obtain copies of these materials, at any time and at no cost, upon request to CVHP.

8.10 **Confidentiality of Arbitration; Survival.** Except as otherwise required by laws, any arbitration resolved pursuant to this Section, including the terms of any final award, shall be confidential. This ARTICLE VIII shall survive termination of this Agreement.

ARTICLE IX
GENERAL PROVISIONS

9.1 **Assignment.** Except as otherwise expressly provided herein, this Agreement may not be assigned by Physician whether voluntarily or by operation of law without the prior written consent of CVHP which may be withheld at CVHP's sole discretion. This Agreement may be assigned by CVHP, upon notice to Physician, to any other person or entity. Subject to the foregoing, this Agreement shall inure to the benefit of and be binding upon the parties hereto and their respective successors and permitted assigns. Any attempted assignment in contravention of this Section shall be void.

9.2 **Attorney's Fees.** In the event of any action or proceeding brought by either party against the other under this Agreement, including, without limitation, arbitration, the prevailing party shall be entitled to recover from the other party all of its reasonable costs and expenses, including without limitation, the reasonable fees and costs of its attorneys.

9.3 **Authority.** This Agreement constitutes the legal, valid, and binding obligation of the parties. Each party represents and warrants that it has the right, power, authority, and capacity to execute and deliver this Agreement and to perform its respective obligations under this Agreement.

9.4 **Binding Agreement.** This Agreement has been duly executed and delivered by each party and is the legal, valid, and binding obligation of each party, fully enforceable against each party in accordance with the terms contained herein. Neither CVHP nor Physician is party to any contract, agreement, or obligation that would prevent or hinder it from entering into this Agreement or performing its duties hereunder; nor is any approval or consent of any person, firm, or other entity required to be obtained for the authorization or execution of this Agreement or the performance of duties hereunder.

9.5 **Books and Records.** Physician shall cooperate fully with CVHP by maintaining and making available all necessary records, or by executing any agreements, in order to assure that CVHP will be able to meet all requirements for participation and payment associated with public or private third-party payment programs including, but not limited to, the Medicare and Medicaid programs. Consistent with the foregoing, Physician shall comply with § 1861(v)(1)(I) of the Social Security Act, as amended, and any regulations promulgated pursuant thereto, under which Physician shall maintain its books, documents and records that are necessary to certify the nature and extent of such services and payments under this Agreement and to furnish such books, documents and records, upon written request to the Secretary of Health and Human services or to the Comptroller General, or any of their duly authorized representatives. If Physician is requested to disclose books, documents, or records pursuant to this Section for purpose of an audit, Physician shall notify CVHP of the nature and scope of such request and Physician shall make available, upon written request of CVHP, all such books, documents, or records, during CVHP's regular business hours. This Section shall survive the termination or expiration of this Agreement.

9.6 **Captions.** Any captions to or headings of the articles, sections, subsections, paragraphs, or subparagraphs of this Agreement are solely for the convenience of the parties, are not a part of this Agreement, and shall not be used for the interpretation or determination of validity of this Agreement or any provision hereof.

9.7 **Compliance with Laws.** At all times during the duration of this Agreement, each party shall comply in all material respects: (i) with all applicable laws, including, without limitation, 42 U.S.C. Section 1320a-7b (the "**Anti-kickback Statute**") and the federal physician self-referral law set forth at 42 I.S.C. Section 1395nn and all related regulations (the "**Stark law**"), all similar state laws and all Federal health care program requirements, and (ii) with all of CVHP's and/or each Facility's policies and procedures, protocols, bylaws rules and regulations, as applicable, and Physician shall anticipate in any training relating to the Anti-kickback Statute and the Stark law. Physician shall provide CVHP with any certifications CVHP may reasonable request from time to time to memorialize Physician's agreement to comply with the terms of this Section 9.7.

9.8 **Counterparts.** This Agreement may be executed in counterparts, each of which shall be deemed an original, but all of which together shall constitute but one and the same agreement.

9.9 **Entire Agreement; Amendment.** This Agreement contains the entire agreement of the parties hereto and supersedes all prior agreements, contracts and understandings, whether written or otherwise, between the parties relating to the subject matter hereof. This Agreement or any provision hereof may be modified or amended only by mutual written agreement of the parties. Any such modification or amendment must be in writing, dated and signed by the parties and attached to this Agreement.

9.10 **Exclusivity.** Physician shall be free to perform professional services for other patients and entities outside of CVHP, and nothing in this Agreement shall be construed to prohibit Physician from maintaining a separate practice.

9.11 **Exhibits Incorporated by Reference.** The attached attachments, exhibits, and schedules constitute a material part of this Amendment and are to be construed as incorporated in this Amendment and are made a part hereof.

9.12 **Governing Law; Venue.** The validity, interpretation, and performance of this Agreement shall be governed by and construed in accordance with the laws of the State of California, without regard to its conflicts of laws principles. The venue for any judicial proceeding brought by either party with regard to any provision of or obligation arising under this Agreement shall be in Los Angeles County, California.

9.13 **Health Information Privacy.** Each party hereto shall perform its duties and obligations hereunder in a manner consistent with applicable federal and state laws governing the privacy and security of patient information, including, without limitation, the Health Insurance Portability ad Accountability Act of 1996 and the rules and regulations promulgated thereunder ("**HIPAA**"), the Health Information Technology for economic and Clinical Health Act of 2009 and the rules and regulations promulgated thereunder ("**HITECH**"), the California Confidentiality of Medical Information act, Cal. Civ. Code Section 56 et seq. ("**CMIA**"), and the California Patient Access to Health Records Act, Cal. Health & Saf. Code Section 123100 et seq. ("**PAHRA**"), as the same may be amended from time to time. CVHP is a "covered entity," as such term is defined under HIPAA. If requested by CVHP during the term of the Agreement, Physician shall participate in an Organized Health Care Arrangement ("**OHCA**") with CVHP and comply with CVHP's OHCA-related policies, procedures, and notice of privacy practices under HIPAA.

9.14 **Litigation Consultation.** Physician shall not knowingly accept consulting assignments or otherwise contract, agree or enter into an engagement to provide expert testimony or evaluation on behalf of a plaintiff in connection with any claim asserting negligence, malpractice or professional liability on the part of CVHP, or any subsidiary or affiliate thereof is named, or expected to be named, as a defendant.

9.15 **No Third-Party Beneficiaries.** The obligations created by this Agreement shall be enforceable only by the parties hereto, and no provision of this Agreement is intended, nor shall any provision be construed, to create any rights for the benefit of, or enforceable by any third persons. This Agreement is not intended, nor shall it be construed, to establish any duties or standard of care with respect to any third person.

9.16 **Notices.** Any notices required or permitted to be given hereunder by either party to the other shall be given in writing, by personal delivery, by overnight delivery service, or by registered or certified mail. Postage prepaid, with return receipt requested, or by e-mail. Notices shall be addressed to the applicable party at the address appearing below, or to such other place as the party may from time to time designate in writing to the other party in accordance with this Section. Notices delivered personally shall be deemed to have been received at the time of delivery; notices delivered by overnight mail shall be deemed to have been received 1 day after proper delivery of the notice to the overnight delivery service; mailed notices shall be deemed to have been received as of 3 days after mailing; notices delivered via e-mail shall be deemed to have been received upon e-mail confirmation of receipt.

If to CVHP: Citrus Valley Health Partners
210 W. San Bernardino Road
Covina, CA 91723
Attn: Chief Executive Officer

If to Physician: ______________________
____
____
____
Attn: ______________________

9.1 **Remedies.** The remedies provided in this Agreement are cumulative and are in addition to any other remedies in law or equity which may be available to the non-breaching party in the event of default. The election of one or more remedies shall not bar the use of other remedies unless the circumstances make the remedies incompatible, nor shall it be deemed a waiver of or an election not to assert any other such right or remedy.

9.2 **Severability.** If any provision of this Agreement is held by a court of competent jurisdiction to be invalid, void, or unenforceable, the remaining provisions shall nevertheless continue in full force and effect, unless such construction would defeat an essential purpose of this Agreement.

9.3 **Waiver** Any waiver of any terms and conditions hereof must be in writing, and signed by the parties hereto. Any waiver of any right hereunder in a specific circumstance shall not be deemed a waiver of that right in any other circumstances or a waiver of any other right. To be valid, a waiver must be in writing but need not be supported by consideration.

IN WITNESS WHEREOF, the parties have caused this Agreement to be executed by their duly authorized representatives as of the Effective Date.

"CVHP":	**"PHYSICIAN":**
CITRUS VALLEY HEALTH PARTNERS,	______________________, M.D.
a California non-profit corporation	an individual
By: ______________________	By: ______________________
Print Name: ______________________	Print Name: ______________________
Title: ______________________	

EXHIBIT 1.1
PHYSICIAN COACHING SERVICES

The Services shall include the following:

1. **Assignment of Mentees**. Physician shall provide the Services to such physicians as Physician and CVHP agree from time to time (each a "**Mentee**" and, collectively, "**Mentees**"). CVHP shall maintain a list of Mentees assigned to Physician, which list shall include at least the following information: (a) Mentee's name; (b) date of assignment of Mentee to Physician; and (c) any particular areas of coaching on which CVHP would like Physician to focus with such Mentee. CVHP shall provide the then-current list of mentees to Physician upon Physician's request. Each Physician shall be assigned a maximum of 3 Mentees.
2. **Services**. Physician shall provide the following Services:
    - Meet with each Mentee one cumulative hour per week and provide one-on-one coaching to improve patient satisfaction and enhance physician engagement.
    - Attend the CVHP Leadership Academy. The schedule of classes is listed in Exhibit 1.2.
    - Attend other programs of instruction related to patient satisfaction as mutually agreed by Physician and CVHP.
    - Provide other related services as required or reasonably requested by CVHP.

EXHIBIT 1.2
DRAFT SCHEDULE OF CVHP LEADERSHIP ACADEMY SESSIONS

The following schedule is in draft format and is subject to change. Each Physician must complete one class from each session, for a total of 8 h of class time. These hours will be compensated at the base rate listed in this agreement. Locations will be announced

Session 1-Choose 1 course	• Tuesday June 5, 2012 12:00–2:00 PM • Thursday June 7, 2012 12:00–02:00 PM
Session 2-Choose 1 course	• Thursday June 21, 2012 9:00–11:00 AM • Tuesday June 26, 2012 12:00–2:00 PM
Session 3-Choose 1 course	• Tuesday July 10, 2012 9:00–11;00 AM • Thursday July 12, 2012 12:00–2:00 PM
Session 4-Choose 1 course	• Tuesday July 24 2012 9:00–11:00 AM • Tuesday August 7, 2012 12:00–02:00 PM

EXHIBIT 1.3
FORM OF PHYSICIAN COACHING SERVICES TIME RECORDS
(PLEASE PRINT OR TYPE ALL INFORMATION)

Mentee Name	Coaching Dates	Issues Coached	Time Spent (hours)
Mentee 1-			
Mentee 2-			
Mentee 3-			

EXHIBIT 2.1
COMPENSATION FOR PHYSICIAN COACHING SERVICES

1. **General Principles**. The goal of the Agreement is to appropriately compensate Physician for effectively providing the Services which, as a result, will assist CVHP in developing and maintaining consistently high standards of professionalism across all physicians who provide care to patients at the Facilities. The compensation to be paid by CVHP to Physician pursuant to this Agreement has been established, and any changes in compensation shall be made, in a manner that fairly and appropriately compensates Physician for the reasonable fair market value of the Services provided by Physician hereunder. To reward exceptional results, a portion of the compensation under this Agreement will be tied to the achievement of certain mutually agreed-upon outcomes, as specified more fully below.
2. **Base Compensation**. In exchange for providing the Services, CVHP shall pay Physician a base fee of <u>One Hundred Dollars ($100) per hour</u> (**Base Fee**) CVHP's obligation to pay the Base Fee shall be conditioned on Physician's compliance with the terms set forth in the Agreement, including, without limitation: (i) pursuant to <u>Section 3.2</u>, CVHP's receipt of documentation required under <u>Section 1.6</u> regarding the time spent and nature of the Services provided by contractor during the preceding month, and (ii) the number of Physician's hours of Services shall not exceed <u>12 h per month</u> (**Maximum Monthly Hours**").
3. **Performance Bonus**. In addition to the Base Fee, for each 12 month period following the Effective Date (the "**Performance Bonus Measurement Period**"), Physician shall have the opportunity to earn a performance bonus of up to <u>$14,400</u> ("**Performance Bonus**") based on the achievement of certain mutually agreed performance criteria set forth in <u>Attachment 3.1</u>, attached hereto and incorporated herein by this reference (the "**Performance Bonus Criteria**").

   (a) <u>Updates to Performance Bonus Criteria.</u> The Performance Bonus Criteria may be reviewed and updated by mutual written agreement of CVHP and Physician; provided, however, that the initial Performance Bonus Criteria, and any subsequently updated Performance bonus Criteria, shall remain in place for at least 1 year. Any updates to the Performance Bonus Criteria shall be memorialized in a written amendment to this <u>Exhibit 3.1</u>, signed by CVHP and Physician.

   (b) <u>Timing and Payment of Performance Bonus.</u> The Performance Bonus, if any, shall be calculated at the end of each Performance Bonus Measurement Period, and shall be paid by CVHP to Physician on or before 30 days following the Performance Bonus Measurement Period for which the Performance Bonus was calculated.

4. **Adjustment**. The compensation methodology described herein shall be in effect for the Initial Term, and shall continue thereafter unless changed or modified by the parties.

ATTACHMENT 3.1
BONUS CRITERIA

The quarterly bonus is based on achieving the 51st percentile on the HCAHPS composite score for physician communication in the aggregate for all CVHP inpatient facilities. The first quarterly incentive (for two quarters of up to $7,200) to be paid in January 2013, subject to aggregate physician communication scores for CVHP to be at or above 51st percentile for two quarters ending December 31, 2012.

Subsequently, quarterly incentive of $3,600 per quarter per physician will be paid if aggregate physician communication score for CVHP are at or above 51st percentile during the preceding quarter.

Payout Period	Measurement Period	Maximum Payout
January 2013	July 2012–December 2012	$7,200
April 2013	January 2013–March 2013	$3,600
July 2013	April 2013–June 2013	$3,600

Reviewed and Approved
Facility Administrator

Signature Date

Print Name

Reviewed and Approved By:

Signature Date

Print Name

MD Welcome Letter Sample

Dear Doctor,

Congratulations on your CVHP medical staff leadership position for Year 2015. This is an exciting new year for our organization as we improve our efforts to provide patient centered quality care. We will continue to hold each other accountable as we move to the next level of quality patient care and patient safety. Consequently, our CVHP Transforming the Patient Experience committee has provided you with a free copy of Dr. Marty Makary's book. "Unaccountable."

The book has been read by the executive management team and the CVHP Physician coaches. As a medical staff leader, we believe you will find Dr. Makary's book both illuminating and inspiring. Our goal is to help people keep well in body mind and spirit by providing quality healthcare services in a compassionate environment. Have a great new year.

Sincerely,

Chief Transformation Officer

Physician Care Champions

We frequently recognize the doctors our patients have selected as physician care champions. These men and women exemplify the best in our CVHP family. They give true meaning to our "expectation of excellence" from all who are involved with patient care. As we continue this transformational journey, we will stay committed to help people keep well in body mind and spirit, by providing quality health care services in a compassionate environment.

Chapter 6
Hospital Champions

In March 2013, an example of how to integrate MD leaders occurred. Rob and I were going on our routine pain rounds at one of our hospitals. We stopped by one of the offices of an executive who was finalizing a site visit plan to Sharp Hospital in San Diego, CA. The purpose of the onsite visit was to evaluate a new program we might be interested in that Sharp Hospital was using. The name of the program was First Touch later changed to Building Connections.

It was developed by Lolma Olsen. Lolma is a Clinical Registered Nurse who discovered there was a better way to communicate with and treat patients. Our Sharp Hospital visit was informative, inspiring and motivating. Our group led by Rob our CEO, immediately decided to implement the Building Connections program. The philosophy of Building Connections is to take the best of who we are and connect to the best in the people we serve. It is a transformative program designed to improve quality care and mutual respect (see Fig. 6.1).

W.T. Choctaw, *Transforming the Patient Experience*,
DOI 10.1007/978-3-319-16928-6_6

BUILDING
CONNECTIONS

The *Building Connections* Framework

The Philosophy

Taking the best of who we are and connecting with the best in the people we serve.

Storytelling

Concept	*Concept*	*Concept*
Be Present	**Suspend Judgment**	**Practice Touch**

Process

Hello:	Makes an initial personal connection
	Leave armor behind
	Sit down eye-to-eye, heart-to-heart
Retouch:	Reaffirm your connection
Handoffs:	Smooth the transition, transfer trust
Goodbye:	Meaningful goodbye, transfer trust

Outcomes

- Improves patient experiences and satisfaction
- Enhances collegial relationships
- Reduces patient/family fear and anxiety
- Establishes trust

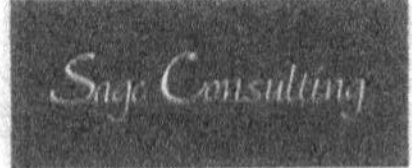

Fig. 6.1 Lolma Olsen's Training Outline

Gold Star Partners 100th Milestone

A historic milestone was reached on January 2014 when the 100th CVHP employee was recognized by CVHP Physician Coaches. Gold star partners are employees who demonstrate exceptional service that helps patients. We believe, all our employees are caregivers whether they work in an office or at the bedside. Each employee determines the patient experience. The Beryl Institute defines the patient experience as "the sum of all interactions, shaped by the organization's culture, that influence patient perceptions, across the continuum of care". These elite high performance individuals are the essence of our transformation as an organization. New gold star partners are identified monthly in the Physician-2-Physician monthly newsletter (see Fig. 6.2).

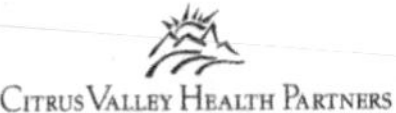

Physicians' Gold Star Partners

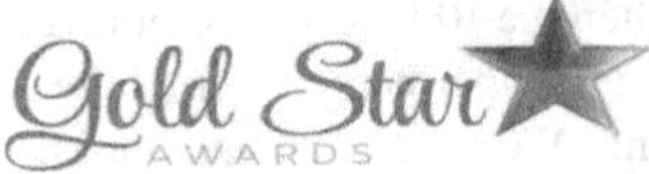

Telesforo Sanchez - Recognized by Dr. Michele Vargas for going above and beyond to ensure the cleanliness of the Emergency Department at FPH.

Danny Espinoza - Recognized by Dr. Subhash Dhand for always working hard to make sure the ICC campus is clean and tidy.

Lolly Henderson, RN, MSN; Lori Bryant; Darlene Coker & Sheryl Claveria, RN - Recognized by Dr. Scott Isbell for working extremely hard on the ED Flow Green Belt Project. Their effort and hard work is already making a difference.

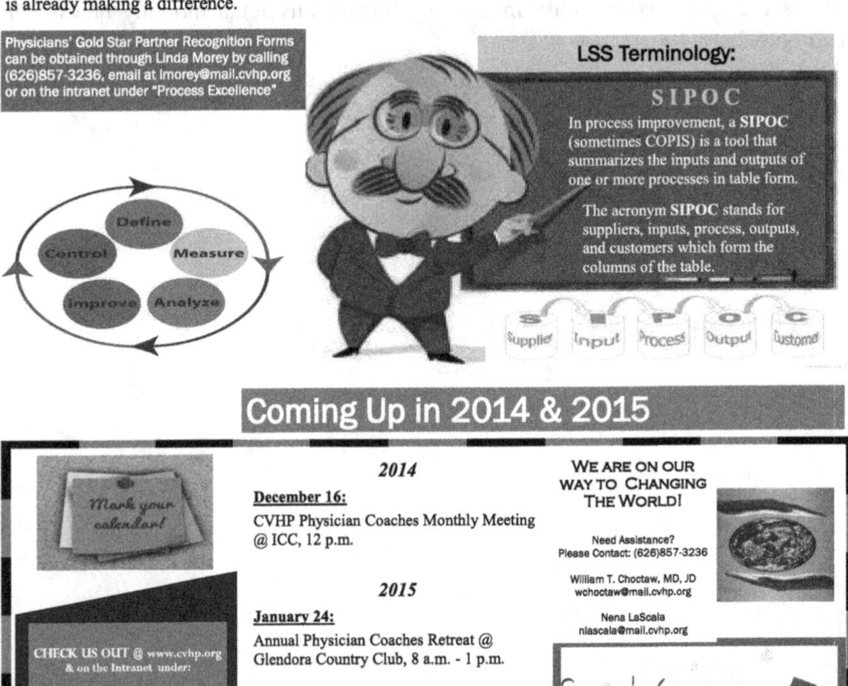

Physicians' Gold Star Partner Recognition Forms can be obtained through Linda Morey by calling (626)857-3236, email at lmorey@mail.cvhp.org or on the intranet under "Process Excellence"
Define
Measure
Analyze
Improve
Control
LSS Terminology:
SIPOC
In process improvement, a SIPOC (sometimes COPIS) is a tool that summarizes the inputs and outputs of one or more processes in table form.
The acronym SIPOC stands for suppliers, inputs, process, outputs, and customers which form the columns of the table.
S I P O C
Supplier Input Process Output Customer

Coming Up in 2014 & 2015

Mark your calendar!

CHECK US OUT @ www.cvhp.org & on the Intranet under:

Process Excellence

2014

December 16:
CVHP Physician Coaches Monthly Meeting @ ICC, 12 p.m.

2015

January 24:
Annual Physician Coaches Retreat @ Glendora Country Club, 8 a.m. - 1 p.m.

Quarterly Physician Building Connections Workshop

February 2, ICC @ 12 p.m.
May 4, Foothill @ 5:30 p.m.
August 3, QVC @ 12 p.m.
November 2, ICC @ 5:30 p.m.

WE ARE ON OUR WAY TO CHANGING THE WORLD!

Need Assistance?
Please Contact: (626)857-3236

William T. Choctaw, MD, JD
wchoctaw@mail.cvhp.org

Nena LaScala
nlascala@mail.cvhp.org

Season's Greetings & Happy New Year

Fig. 6.2 Process Excellence LSS Newsletter

Chapter 7
Lean Six Sigma: The Joint Commission

Robust Process Improvement (RPI) has arrived at CVHP. RPI is change management and Lean Six Sigma. Lean is based on the Toyota system. It is a proven long term approach for engaging people and aligning systems into processes that eliminate waste and deficiencies in the process. Six Sigma was created by Motorola and popularized by General Electric. It deploys a structured; project focused statistical approach to eliminate waste and variability in quality. RPI has a proven sustainability element that allows the changes it creates to be fundamental and irreversible. We have contracted with The Joint Commission (TJC) to provide in house training for our staff and physicians. TJC has assisted many hospitals become highly reliable organizations. We are delighted to have the opportunity to partner with them.

Our partnership with the Center for Transforming Healthcare part of The Joint Commission has been extremely helpful. Here are some comments from Anne Marie Benedicto, Executive Vice President Support Operations and Chief of Staff The Joint Commission about our partnership:

In January 2014, Citrus Valley Health Partners (CVHP) adopted Robust Process Improvement® (RPI®) as part of an on-going system-wide initiative to dramatically improve the efficiency of its internal operations, increase patient satisfaction, and ensure that patient care at CVHP is consistently excellent and consistently safe, RPI®, along with leadership and a strong safety culture, are components of high reliability health care. By learning and using process improvement tools and methods that have been used successfully in health care and in other industries, such as Lean Six Sigma and Change Management, CVHP staff will acquire a common language, skill set and understanding for improvement.

RPI® will be used internally at CVHP to increase organization-wide capacity for improvement. A key goal of the RPI® initiative is to embed use of these tools and methods unto the daily work of the health system and to build the expertise of staff and leadership. A central feature of the initiative is an aggressive training program that features classroom learning coupled with practical application of the RPI® tool set to solve complex problems and improve business operations and clinical

W.T. Choctaw, *Transforming the Patient Experience*,
DOI 10.1007/978-3-319-16928-6_7

outcomes that will positively impact the care experienced by CVHP patients and their families.

One of the many strengths of RPI® is the combination of data-driven problem solving (through Lean Six Sigma) with the change management capability of Facilitating Change™. The inclusion of Facilitating Change™ underscores that a great technical solution is often not enough for sustainability. Recognizing the needs and ideas of the people who are part of the process—and who we are charging with implementing and sustaining a new solution—is important in building buy-in and engagement.

CVHP engaged RPI® experts from the Joint Commission Center for Transforming Healthcare to train staff in RPI® tools and methods. The Center's engagement model has a strong train-the-trainer component, which will help CVHP build a strong internal RPI® program and ensure its sustainability.

At the Joint Commission, we began our own RPI® deployment in 2008, and we use RPI® to improve our products and services and the experience of our customers. RPI® is also the methodology used by the Joint Commission Center for Transforming Healthcare to identify solutions for some of health care's most persistent problems, such as eliminating healthcare-associated infection and wrong-site surgeries. We are pleased to be part of CVHP's high reliability journey.

Frequently Asked Questions About RPI at CVHP

1. What is Robust Process Improvement (RPI)?

RPI is a set of strategies, tools, methods, and training programs adopted by Citrus Valley Health Partners (CVHP) for improving their business processes, operations and clinical outcomes. A process is robust when it consistently achieves high quality in the following ways:

- Defining factors critical to quality
- Using data and data analysis to design improvement
- Enlisting stakeholders and process owners in creating and sustaining solutions
- Eliminating defects and waste
- Drastically decreasing failure rates
- Simplifying and increasing the speed of processes
- Partnering with staff and leaders to seek, commit to, and accept change.

The RPI tool kit includes methodologies that have been proven effective in many sectors, including health care, and have been used to achieve dramatic improvements in clinical and operational quality, in cost savings and in efficiency. These methodologies include Lean Six Sigma and change management. All the tools in the RPI tool kit have strong conceptual underpinnings that drive and sustain positive change, such as the value of an empowered work force, the goal of efficiency, and the desire for excellence.

Lean Six Sigma and Change Management make up the basic "tool kit" within RPI. These methodologies have long histories, each with supporters and detractors. We refer to these methodologies collectively as "Robust Process Improvement" because we recognize the richness of each of these tool sets and the advantage of having a variety of approaches to address opportunities for improvement in the complex environments of hospitals and health systems. Each of the tool sets are explained in detail in the following pages.

Successful adoption of RPI will produce substantial improvements in the efficiency and quality of our internal processes and services, which will translate to patient care that is consistently excellent and consistently safe. The successful deployment of RPI will support and strengthen CVHP's goal to foster a culture of learning and excellence, and gain recognition as a model practitioner of highly effective process improvement.

2. Why is RPI important?

RPI is important because the methodology has the breath, flexibility and analytical strength necessary to address complex, multi-factorial and long-standing patient safety problems.

In 1999, the Institute of Medicine report "To Err is Human" galvanized the health care field on the need to dramatically improve patient safety by reducing preventable errors—some of which result in patient harm.

Fifteen years later, despite widespread attention to improvement, safety issues continue to persist in our health care organizations and they continue to hurt patients. It is clear that new methods of improvement are necessary to produce breakthrough changes to keep patients safe in an increasingly complex health care context.

Many of the most persistent and widespread safety issues in health care—such as wrong site surgery and healthcare-associated infections—are complex and multi-factorial. For many health care organizations, the usual approach to problem solving or process improvement involves looking at others' so-called best practices, protocols, checklists, bundles, or tool kits and then dropping them in your organization. That one-size-fits-all approach only works in limited circumstances—such as when the process varies very little and when the causes of failure are few and common.

We need a problem solving methodology that has the sophistication to handle complex problems, and that can recognize that:

- Failures in health care performance have many causes
- Key causes differ from place to place
- Each cause requires a different strategy to solve
- A set of solutions that works in one facility will not be as effective in another

Therefore, you need a problem solving methodology that allows you to identify your root causes and come up with solutions to address those.

Because RPI allows us to explore complexity, it is effective in addressing the complex, multi-factorial problems such as Hospital Acquired Infections, Hand Washing, and Patient Falls with Injury. It is also appealing to clinicians and other health care workers because of its data driven approach.

Finally, The Joint Commission identified RPI as one of the three components of high reliability health care. Widespread use of RPI within a hospital or hospital system increases that organization's capacity for improvement and is a strong driver of culture change.

3. RPI Deconstructed: What is Six Sigma?

Six Sigma is a statistical model that measures a process in terms of defects. Six Sigma allows an organization to achieve quality by using a set of strategies, tools, and methods designed to improve processes so that less than 3.4 defects (i.e., errors or unexpected or undesired results) exist for every million opportunities. Through the focus Six Sigma methods provide, processes are as close to perfect as possible. Sigma, or the Greek letter δ, is the symbol for standard deviation in statistics, and standard deviation levels help us understand how much the process deviates from perfection.

Six Sigma is also a philosophy of management that emphasizes the following:

- The importance of understanding factors critical to quality and customer expectations
- The measurement and analysis of data
- The implementation of solutions designed to improve processes to affect the most statistically significant sources of variation
- Sustaining these solutions

In short, Six Sigma is several things:

- A statistical basis of measurement that strives for reduction of defects to 3.4 defects per million opportunities (DPMO)
- A data-driven, step-wise, problem-solving methodology that relies on measurement and statistical analysis
- A philosophy and a goal: to be as perfect as practically possible
- A symbol of quality

Motorola started using Six Sigma in the 1980s to improve its manufacturing processes. GE and others expanded Six Sigma's applicability to service processes with great success. Other users and innovators in the late 1990s include DuPont, Dow Chemical, 3M, Ford, Amex, Bank of America, JP Morgan Chase, and United Health Care. (From Six Sigma for Managers, G. Brue, 2002)

4. RPI Deconstructed: What is Lean?

Lean is a well-defined set of tools that increase customer value by eliminating waste and creating flow throughout the value stream. The following describes lean improvement:

- Inexpensive to implement
- Focus on improving processes, not people
- Address the batch and queue mentality of silos by following process flow
- Promote simple, error-proof systems

Therefore, a lean process is better (because it has no defects and reflects what the customer wants), cheaper (because non-value added work is removed and there is no re-work or scrap), and faster (because it eliminates batch and queue, introduces flow, and gets it right the first time).

The Lean Steps:

- Specify Value—from the customer's perspective
- Map the Process—Process Map or Value Stream Map
- Identify Value Added and Non-Value Added Steps
- Examine Flow—continuous, minimally interrupted flow; single piece vs. batching
- Create Pull—do not produce until the next step downstream is ready for you
- Pursue Perfection—sustain improvement; change culture

5. RPI Deconstructed: What is Lean Six Sigma?

Recognizing the complementary nature of the two methodologies, many organizations have used Lean and Six Sigma concurrently, utilizing different pieces of the tool kit to address specific improvement problems along a value stream. This practice of combining different tool sets and playing to strengths is called a "blended approach." CVHP's blended approach has Lean Six Sigma, as well as Facilitating Change and Work Out.

6. RPI Deconstructed: What is change management?

Change management is a set of actions, supported by a tool set, used to prepare an organization to seek, commit to, and accept change. Change management tools increase the exposure and participation of staff and leadership in shaping new solutions and interventions. These tools increase the speed in which the proposed change is adapted and accepted and reinforce its effectiveness.

The model we used for change management is called Facilitating Change. The Facilitating Change Model has four components with important activities within each that describe what is necessary to most effectively transition an organization from its current state to the desired improved state:

- Plan Your Project
- Inspire People
- Launch the Initiative
- Support the Change

Facilitating Change is the change management model created by The Joint Commission, recognizing that the need to direct constant change is critical to any dynamic business environment, and is especially true in health care.

7. How will RPI affect my work?

The use of RPI in the daily work of Citrus Valley is the ultimate goal of RPI deployment and is a sign that improvement is fully embedded into the organization's culture.

RPI is about process improvement, and as we learn the tools of RPI, you and your colleagues will use the tool set to improve your processes for your organization and the patients you serve. Your department may be involved in a project led by Black Belts, or Green Belts, or you may be asked to participate in the many groups and teams that will inform the work of that Black Belt and Green Belts. We invite you to learn about the project's goals and share ideas about how to make your processes more robust.

You should consider taking advantage of RPI training and certification opportunities that will soon be available. In addition you should start thinking about improvement opportunities in your area that might make your life easier or have a positive impact on patient care. When improvement teams start forming, volunteer to join one of them, or participate in the project progress reports or repot-outs.

8. If the goal is for the entire health system to utilize RPI concepts in our daily work, how will that come to fruition if only a few select people get the in-depth training?

Although the full breadth and rigor of the training process make ti impossible for all employees to be trained at once, leadership envisions some level of Lean Six Sigma and change management training for all employees. Our strategy is to seed the organization with trained staff that will use their skills while working with their colleagues, thus spreading enthusiasm and establishing a comfort level with RPI methods throughout the health system. The use of RPI as a strategy to achieve improvement goals will proliferate within CVHP as more and more people are trained formally or experience RPI through practical application.

The various training options and deliberate use of RPI methods ensure that CVHP employees have a common language and understanding of improvement, no matter the level of training and exposure.

9. Can anyone be selected for training?

We will begin our first class of Green Belts in the summer of 2014, and additional classes will be held in the future. These training opportunities will be posted and you are encouraged to identify yourself as a candidate if you feel you fit the job description.

10. What are the selection criteria for staff interested in becoming a green Belt or Yellow Belt?

Successful Green Belt trainees are:

- **Skilled change agents**. They have a desire to achieve breakthrough results and expect and know how to manage resistance.
- **Analytical**. They are comfortable with statistics and base their recommendations on data.
- **Passionate about improvement**. They see the possibilities of an improved future state, and are willing to do the work of get there.

- **Leaders**. Each Green Belt trainee will lead an improvement phase. This means organizing the initiative and coordinating with stakeholders and process owners to ensure that the project continues to move forward. The ideal Green Belt trainee has already been recognized as a leader within the organization.
- **Team players**. Green Belt trainees recognize that complex problems are likely to have complex causes which require multiple perspectives. The Green Belt will have the skill to manage team dynamics and strive for a positive outcome. On average, Green Belt project work will take about 25 % of a trainee's time.

11. If I apply to the Green Belt training program and am not selected, can I learn why I was not chosen?

Of course. We expect to have more applicants than training slots—especially in the first training class. Even if you are not selected the first time you apply, we hope you stay interested and apply for future training opportunities.

12. How will staff be empowered through the RPI initiative?

Empowerment is a cornerstone of the methodologies in the RPI tool kit and is critical to the success of RPI deployment. Project teams rely on the participation of a cross section of people closest to a process to generate the best ideas to solve a problem, and to then implement these solutions. Green Belts and Black Belts follow specific steps to identify solutions that are driven by data analysis, stakeholder participation, and customer satisfaction. Lean principles focus on simplifying and error-proofing processes. In a lean environment, you are expected and encouraged to constantly find ways to improve work processes, and then to initiate improvement Facilitating Change tools are designed to increase participation in generating ideas and solutions, build consensus quickly, strengthen accountability and ownership, and support change initiatives.

We will use RPI tools to make decisions and drive improvement by eliciting the expertise and experience. The tools also build accountability by creating the expectation of response and sponsorship from leadership. The tools are not used to force a predetermined solution.

Empowerment begins through learning and through practice. Through our growing RPI expertise, we will have the ability to quickly and effectively address the improvement opportunities we identify. The use of RPI as a strategy to achieve improvement goals, as well as our comfort level with decision making at many different levels of the organization, will increase within CVHP as more and more people are trained formally or experience RPI through practical application.

It is also important to note that successful RPI deployment strengthens an organization's safety culture. Those who actively participate in improvement efforts, identify improvement opportunities, and safety hazards are the hallmark of a safety culture. RPI provides the skills and expertise to act on the improvement opportunities identified.

13. What is DMAIC?

DMAIC is an acronym for Define, Measure, analyze, Improve and Control It is the core of Six Sigma methodology and describes its problem-solving sequence. Here is a short description of the 5 DMAIC steps:

- Define the work to be done and what is critical to quality from the point of view of the sponsor, customer, and stakeholders
- Measure the baseline performance or competitive current state
- Analyze what we need to do differently by identifying the elements that most significantly affect the variability of a process
- Improve the current state by designing interventions that directly address the most significant sources of variation (identified in the Analyze phase)
- Control the process for sustained gains

14. How can RPI be used to improve patient care?

RPI can be used to address any problem, and is particularly suited to the complexity of health care. While many of the methodologies within RPI have been proven effective if addressing business processes and operational issues, many health care organizations have used RPI to successfully and dramatically improve patient care by focusing on persistent, long term patient safety and health care quality issues such as the elimination of health care-associated infections, pain management, improving patient satisfaction, improving core measure performance, eliminating wrong site surgeries, increasing the effectiveness of hand-off communications, and others.

15. What is a report-Out?

A report-out is a structured meeting created for project teams to share their progress with the organization. Green Belt training project teams will do report-outs after each of the five phases of Define, Measure, Analyze, Improve, and Control (or some combination of these).

16. Are there any risks with RPI?

The only risk is not launching RPI. CVHP is committed to providing cost-effective, high-quality health care. Current changes in health care financing means that we have to do more with less reimbursement. We show our commitment to our patients by using our resources effectively and efficiently.

Like every business, we have competitors and cost constraints. The need for continuous improvement is always present and increases every year.

17. What is my role in RPI?

RPI is about process improvement Your role is to learn to use the different tools in the RPI took kit, and then start using these tools every day to improve your daily work processes.

18. How do we know that RPI is successful?

There are many indicators of RPI success. These include the success of RPI projects; the experience of the RPI-trained staff; the increasing use of RPI tools and methods in daily work, and the achievement of the financial goals related to RPI that are set by leadership. To view our comments about our experience with the Joint Commission Center for Transforming Healthcare, visit https://www.dropboxcom/s/705o5dg4f8gdfh/cvhp%20Reliability%20.mp4?d1=0.

Robust Process Improvement Training: First Steps

Structure

- Program Sponsor—Curry
- Engagement Sponsor—Choctaw
- Senior Executive Team—Leadership Tools (Support system, communication, alleviation of barriers)
    - Executive Training for 16 h
    - Black Belt—Choctaw
    - Black Belt—Ronquillo
    - Select 21 Green Belt Candidates (3 weeks training)
    - Determine Number of Projects/Green Belt

Next Steps

- Face to Face Meeting (set expectations)
- Sign Contract
- Set Engagement Date (consider July, August)
- Begin List of Projects (most difficult)
- Biweekly Meetings—Curry Choctaw (June)
- Preliminary Evaluation of ER Flow as RPI Project (May)

My RPI Journey

by

William T. Choctaw, MD

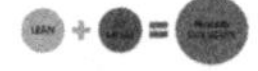

1

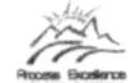

Fig. 7.1 LSS Project Certification Presentation

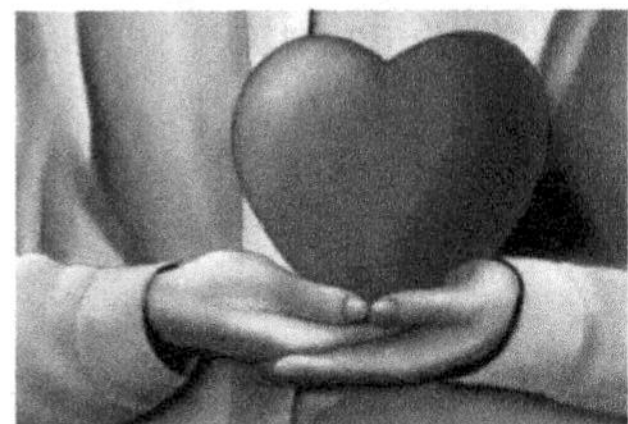

Our CVHP Mission

"TO HELP PEOPLE KEEP WELL IN BODY MIND AND SPIRIT BY PROVIDING QUALITY HEALTHCARE SERVICES IN A SAFE AND COMPASSIONATE ENVIRONMENT"

2

Fig. 7.1 (continued)

Effective Hand-Off Communication Between QVC ED and QVC DOU3

Green Belt Team:
Angela Bernacki
Lourdes Casao, RN
William Choctaw, MD
Tracy Dallarda
Sponsor: Rob Curry
Champion: Melissa Howard, RN
Process Owner: Gem Lindsay, RN
Process Owner: Diane Freeman, RN
Process Owner: Kathi Hemphill, RN

March 19, 2015

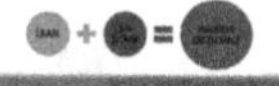

3

Fig. 7.1 (continued)

The Green Belt Team

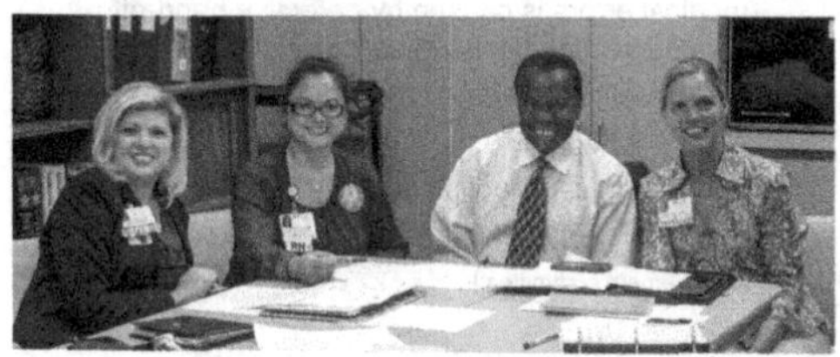

Change Management

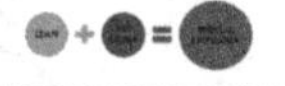

4

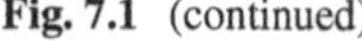

Fig. 7.1 (continued)

Define

- SMART
- 15 Words
- Charter
- Stakeholder Analysis
- Fist of 5
- Circle of Influence/ Circle of Control
- Kano Analysis
- SIPOC

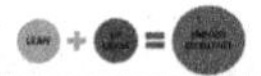

5

Fig. 7.1 (continued)

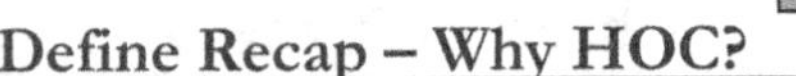

Define Recap – Why HOC?

- Problem & Voice of Customer
  - The Joint Commission concluded 80% of serious medical errors is caused by defective hand-off communication between caregivers
  - Our Baseline defective rate 38% is high (targeted solutions tool)
  - Low patient satisfaction scores (Press Ganey), high number of sentinel events (CVHP quality performance improvement committee)

"It is in inadequate hand-offs that safety often fails first."
-Institute of Medicine

6

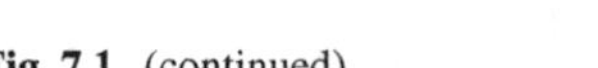

Fig. 7.1 (continued)

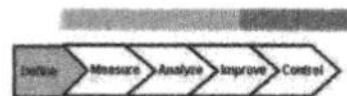

Mission Alignment Case

- Why is it important to CVHP? Our mission is about a

Culture of Safety

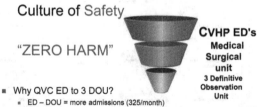

"ZERO HARM"

CVHP ED's Medical Surgical unit 3 Definitive Observation Unit

- Why QVC ED to 3 DOU?
  - ED – DOU = more admissions (325/month)
  - QVC busiest ED in system (X3 size)

Improve processes for effective HOC between Queen of Valley Campus ED & 3 DOU

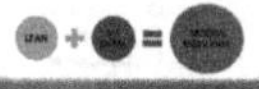

7

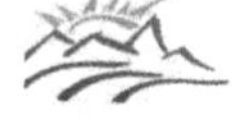

Fig. 7.1 (continued)

Goal

- Primary goal is to reduce the defective hand-off rate by 25% of the baseline defective percentage rate by year end 2014, equivalent to a 28% defective rate
- Secondary goal is to reduce the defective hand-off rate even further, by 50% of baseline defective percentage rate by July 2015
- 1-proportion test in Minitab showed targeted 25% reduction from 38% baseline was statistically significant with $p < 0.05$

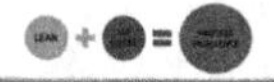

8

Fig. 7.1 (continued)

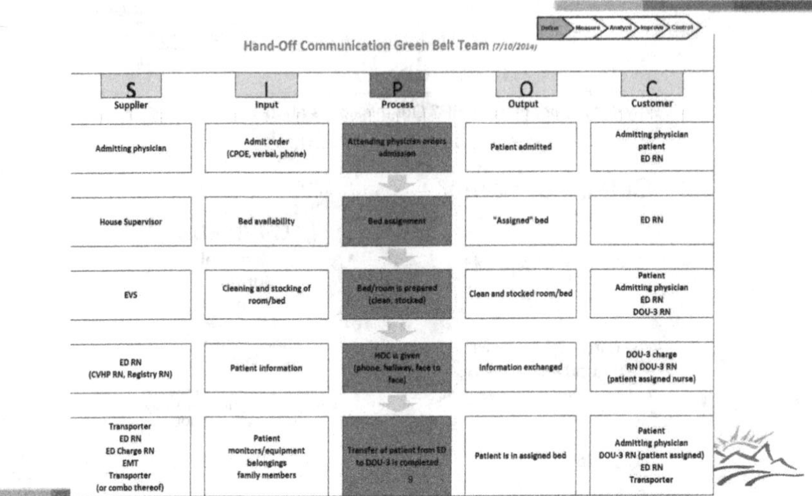

Fig. 7.1 (continued)

Measure & Analyze

- Gemba Walk
- Targeted Solutions Tool
- Data Collection Plan
- Operational Definition
- Measurement Systems Analysis
- Bar Graph
- Pie Graph
- Control chart: p-chart for discreet data

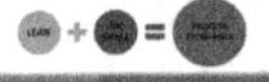

10

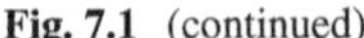

Fig. 7.1 (continued)

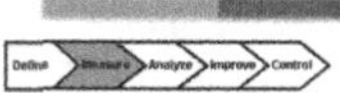

Measure Phase Recap

Data Collection Plan

- Data Collectors: Discreet Data
  - Trained 55 data collectors using tst training module
  - 25 Senders and 30 Receivers were trained
  - Had to pass test with a 90% or above on test before they could become a data collector
- Data collection period: August 20 – October 20
- Collected 120 surveys for baseline

Fig. 7.1 (continued)

Survey Tools – Voice of Process

Hand-off Communication Tool-SENDER

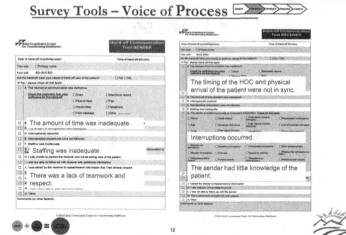

- The amount of time was inadequate.
- Staffing was inadequate.
- There was a lack of teamwork and respect.

Hand-off Communication Tool-RECEIVER

- The timing of the HOC and physical arrival of the patient were not in sync.
- Interruptions occurred.
- The sender had little knowledge of the patient.

12

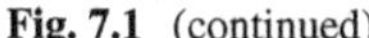

Fig. 7.1 (continued)

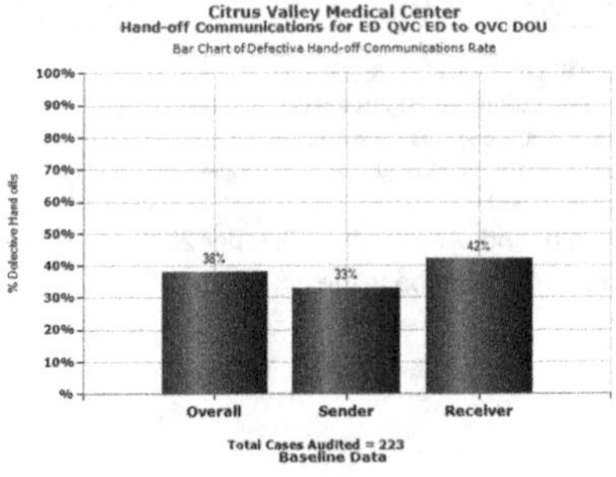

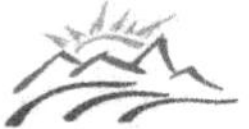

Fig. 7.1 (continued)

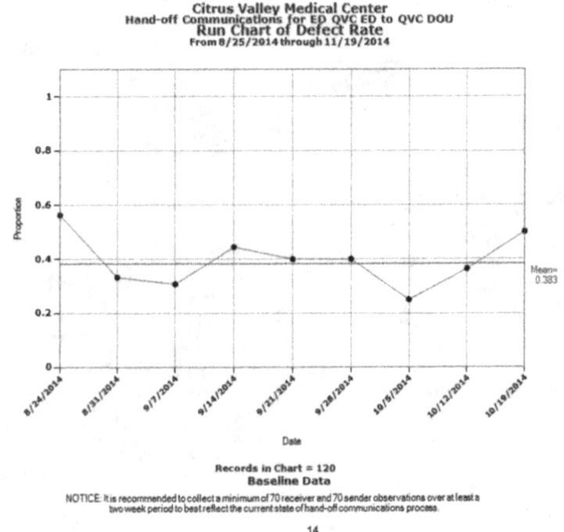

Fig. 7.1 (continued)

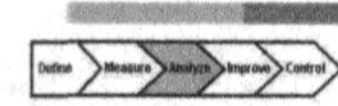

Top 5 Contributing Factors
Baseline Data

Defect	Percent
Inaccurate/incomplete info	21.7%
Knowledge of sender	11.2%
Interruptions	10.5%
Other	9.1%
Information not available Lack of Teamwork/Respect	8.4% 7.0%
Percent overall	***67.9%***

15

Fig. 7.1 (continued)

Improve *& Control*

- 2- Proportion Test
- DFMEA
- SPC Chart
- Process Owner

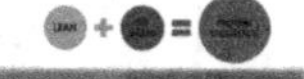
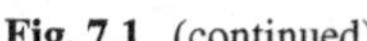

16

Fig. 7.1 (continued)

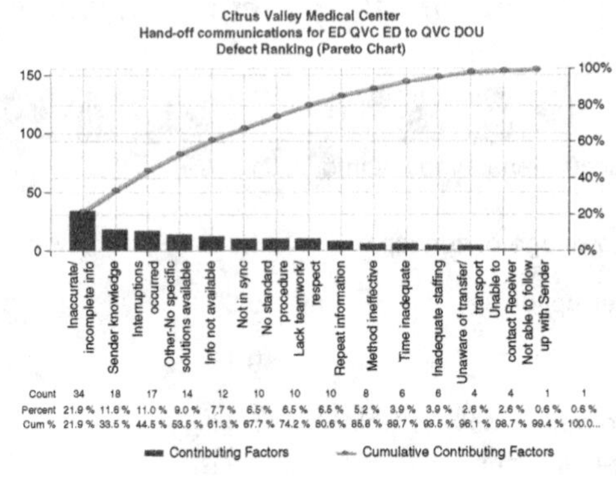

Observations with Defects = 71
Baseline and Improve Data

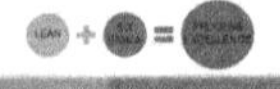

17

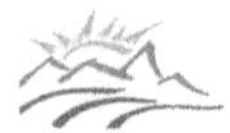

Fig. 7.1 (continued)

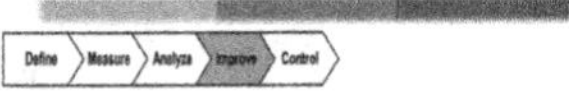

Improvement Phase Recap

- October 21- February 8 improve period. Collected 103 surveys
- Information quality and quantity were root causes
- Customized, standardized SBAR form created
- Education of clinical RN's in the QVC ED and 3 DOU on operational definition of effective HOC
- Improved collaboration and communication between nursing teams

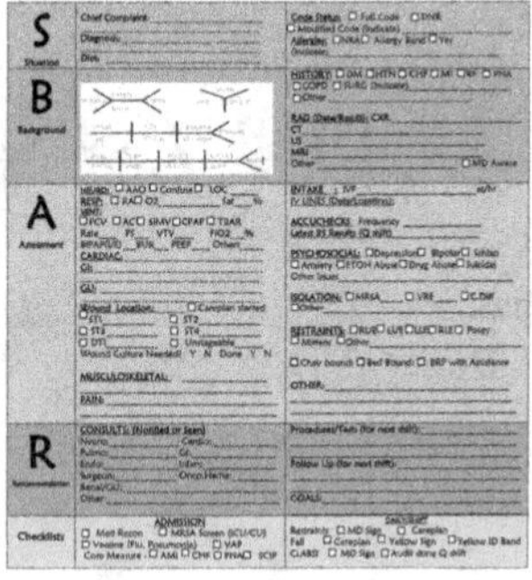

18

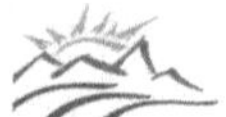

Fig. 7.1 (continued)

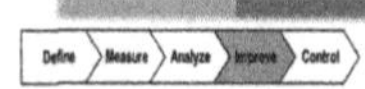

Improvements Made 3/1/15:

- Identification of need for higher frequency of face to face communication when critical patients are being handed off.
- Paper **SBAR** form is being converted to electronic format to be completed within next 30 days.
- Collaboration between nursing teams to improve use of patient bed **Tracker** system is occurring. Tracker training with consultant 3/15.
- **Spectra Link Phones,** have arrived for QVC ED nurses and will be spread to all campuses, to decrease interruptions.

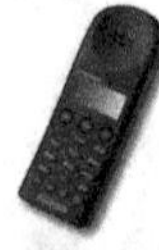

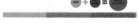

19

Fig. 7.1 (continued)

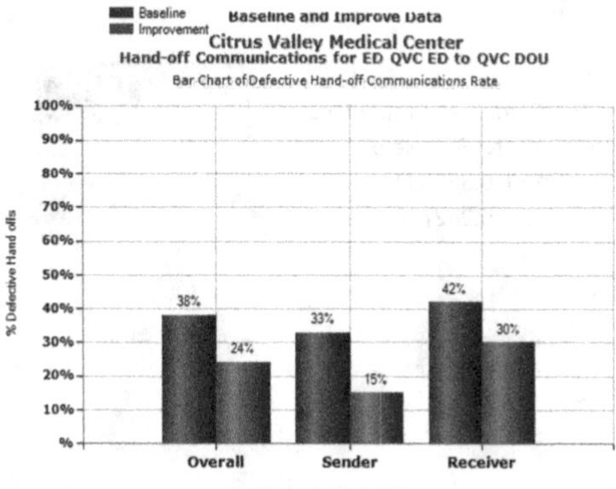

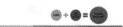

20

Fig. 7.1 (continued)

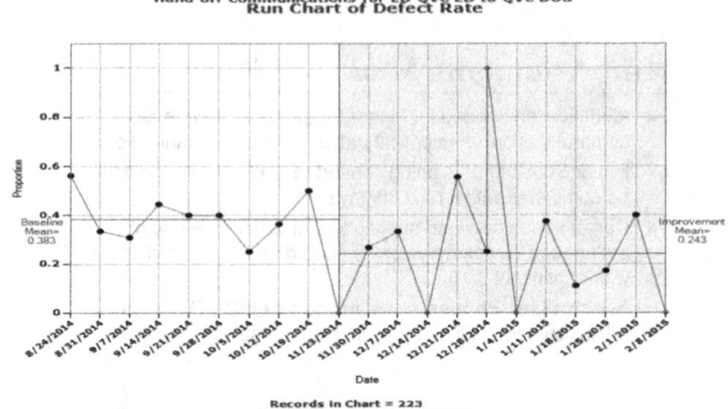

Baseline and Improve Data

NOTICE: It is recommended to collect a minimum of 70 receiver and 70 sender observations over at least a two week period to best reflect the current state of hand-off communications process.

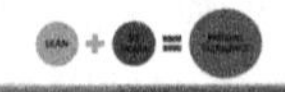

21

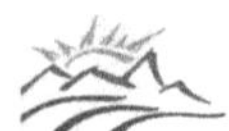

Fig. 7.1 (continued)

Statistical Validation

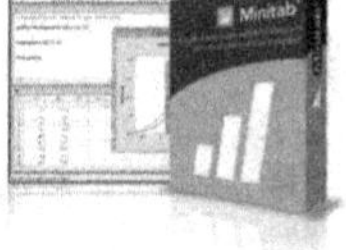

- Test and CI for Two Proportions
- Sample X N Sample p
- 1 46 120 0.383333
- 2 25 103 0.242718

"We reject the Null Hypothesis"

- P-Value = 0.022

"HOC goal was a defective rate decrease to 28% (25% from baseline) on 12/14; Actual statistically validated goal reached was a defective rate decrease to 24% (37% from baseline) on 2/15"

22

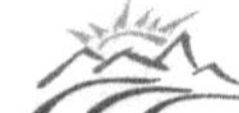

Fig. 7.1 (continued)

Design Failure Modes and Effects Analysis *(DFMEA)*

Process Step	Potential Failure Mode	Potential Failure Effects	SEV	Potential Causes	OCC	Current Process Controls to Prevent Failure Mode	Current Process Controls to Detect Failure Mode	DET	RPN	Recommended Actions	Person Responsible for Actions	Target Completion Date	Actions Taken	New SEV	New OCC	New DET	New RPN
SBAR	Not Used in ER	Increase HOC Defect	9	Nurse apathy	9	Process owner to monitor	Monthly surveys	7	567	Process owner support	Process owner	30 days	Black Belt Coaching	9	7	5	315
	Decrease # of Forms	Increase HOC Defect	9	Unit secretary not monitoring per levels closely	8	Secretary to monitor closely	Weekly surveys	7	504	Educate all secretaries	Unit secretaries	30 days	Training	9	7	4	252
	Not Used in 3 DOU	Increase HOC Defect	9	Nurse apathy	9	Process owner to monitor	Montly surveys	7	567	Process owner support	Process owner	30 days	Black Belt Coaching	9	7	6	378
Tracker	Failure to use properly	Decrease Tracker Usage	8	Decrease knowledge and decrease trust	8	Tracker training	Monthly surveys	9	576	Tracker system manager	Charge nurse	60 days	Bed manager	7	7	8	392
Phone	None available/not in place	Increase HOC Defect	7	Budget	7	Roger Sharma	Monthly Audit	7	343	Acquire phone system	Process owner	5 months	Make quality care	5	8	4	160
Immediate feedback to process owners	Late feedback regarding defective HOC	Increased in HOC defect	9	Interruptions	7	Survey	Review survey, send to process owner within 24 hours	4	252	Contact process owner	Process owner with Black Belt Support	Immediate within 24 hours	Black Belt Coaching	7	7	2	98

Note:

- NOT using the SBAR has high severity of failure and high occurrence
- Opportunity to train and properly use the Tracker communication system could improve HOC and decrease potential failures with information exchange
- Use of Spectra Link Phones will increase the quality and quantity of HOC information and decrease interruptions

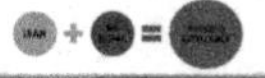

23

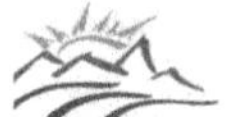

Fig. 7.1 (continued)

Control Plan

Define > Measure > Analyze > Improve > Control

Control Plan											
Project:	Hand Off Communication							Date (Original):		11-Dec-14	
Key Contact:								Date (Revised):		13-Jan-15	
Core Team:	Angela Bernacki, William Choctaw, Tracy Dallarda, Lourdes Casao										
Process Name	Process Step	Input Variable	Output Variable	Process Specification (LSL, USL, Time, Target)	Measurement System Description	MSA Capacity	Fail-Safe Control Method or Monitoring Method	Sample Size	Sample Frequency	Person Responsible for Control	Corrective action
Hand Off Communication	Face to face report	X		25%	Survey	90-100%	Survey	25	Monthly	Unit Directors	Defective rate above 20% Validate root cause for targeted solutions
Hand Off Communication	Telephone report	X		75%	Survey	90-100%	Survey	25	Monthly	Unit Directors	Defective rate above 20% Validate root cause for targeted solutions
Hand Off Communication	Gathering patient information	X		100%	Survey	90-100%	Survey	25	Monthly	Unit Directors	Defective rate above 20% Validate root cause for targeted solutions

24

Fig. 7.1 (continued)

Next Steps:

Who	What	When
HOC Team	Development of Electronic SBAR	March 2015
HOC Team, ED and DOU3 leaders	Official hand off to process owner – Director of critical units QVC	Completed
HOC Team and selected "Spread" leaders	HOC project spread to Foothill Presbyterian Hospital	Completed
Gem Lindsay, Director critical care QVC, **Process Owner**	**Lean Project**: Replacing reusable ECG lead wires with disposable wires at CVHP	Completed

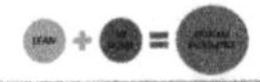

25

Fig. 7.1 (continued)

PROCESS OWNER/SPREAD

- Continue to collect survey data monthly. **3 Process owners** have received all data and are presently getting TST credentials to input data.
- Implement immediate improvements when identified by survey information.
- Coordinate with LSS **Black Belts** and monitor process with statistical process control charts.
- **Green Belt Coaches** are available to assist process owners.
- March 6, 2015- Orientation training began with ER and SICU nurses on HOC project at **FPH.** The **Champion** will be Director of Nursing Education. She will have Black Belt assistance.

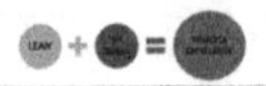

26

Fig. 7.1 (continued)

Thank You!

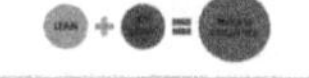

Fig. 7.1 (continued)

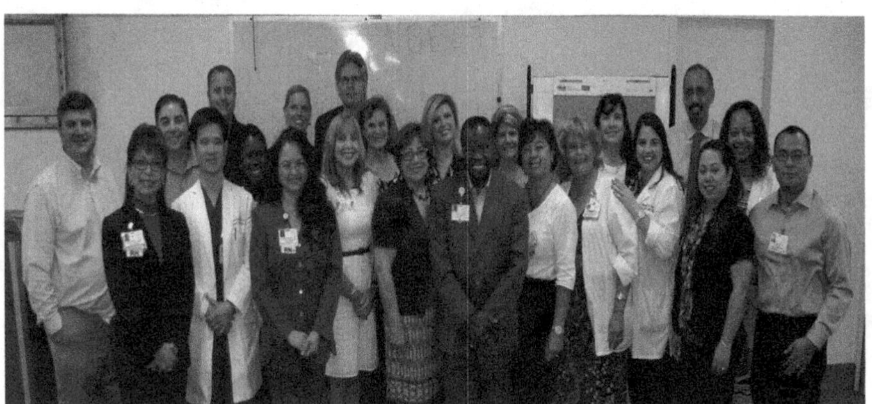

Fig. 7.2 Wave I Lean Six Sigma Green Belts with Black Belt instructors Klaus Nether and Brian Patterson

Chapter 8
Process Excellence

After we had decided to use Lean Six Sigma (LSS) methodology to improve our process, we had to decide where Rapid Process Improvement (RPI)/LSS would fit within our organizational corporate structure. We checked around and noted different approaches by various hospitals. Basically, it was deciding whether the lean six sigma area should be under our traditional performance improvement department or not. Here again, Rob's bold leadership and courage were invaluable. He decided lean six sigma should be implemented at CVHP, system wide at a transformational level. He created a full time executive position, Chief Transformation Officer (CTO) that reports directly to him. The CTO is responsible for developing, implementing and coordinating all robust process improvement lean six sigma activity. Simultaneously, he created an executive cost center and a department we call "Process Excellence."

In the last 8 months, with the Joint Commission, we have trained 21 certified Lean Six Sigma Green Belts (wage 1) including four physicians. They have completed six projects with statistically validated improvements ($p<0.05$). The projects are the following:

1. **Care Continuum**—Heart failure all causes readmission rate decreased from 23 % to 16.7 %.
2. **Emergency Room (ED) Flow**—A reduction in leaving without being seen (LWBS) rate from 3.3 % to 1.5 %. A 50 % decrease in patient wait times to 64 min.
3. **Nurse Handoff Communication**—A decrease in defective rate from 38.3 % to 24.2 %.
4. **Medicare Denial Prevention**—An increase in Physician (2-midnight rule) documentation from 0 % to 56 %. Savings of $443,428 for 1 month.

Electronic supplementary material The online version of this chapter (doi:10.1007/978-3-319-16928-6_8) contains supplementary material, which is available to authorized users.

W.T. Choctaw, *Transforming the Patient Experience*,
DOI 10.1007/978-3-319-16928-6_8

5. **Meditech**—An increase in the electronic submission rate or perinatal measures from 61 % to 91 %.
6. **Surgical Site Infection**—A decrease Surgical Site Infection (SSI) from 22 in 2013 to 11 in 2014. Also, improvement in appropriate dosing of antibiotics by physicians.

The work on all six above projects has been successfully turned over to process owners who will continue the projects as a part of their normal work, creating sustainability. These process owners have been involved with the projects from the beginning as part of the project support team. Additionally, there are many smaller Lean projects that eliminate waste and provide continuous improvement daily. These projects add to the sustainability of our Process Excellence program by providing a broader foundation for our Green Belts.

Finally, our process excellence initiative is exemplary of the early stage of our clinical integration with our physicians. In 2014 physicians constituted 20 % of the 21 Lean Six Sigma Green Belts. In 2015, physicians will be 25 % of the 26 Green Belts. I am the Deployment Leader for our Lean Six Sigma program and active member of our medical staff. I am also a Black Belt member of our CVHP executive team.

Chapter 9
Summary

This book shares a part of CVHP's journey to transform the patient experience. It begins with the premise that although transformation begins with the person in the mirror, it can be developed, launched and implemented with the smallest team possible—2 people. Two people who are leaders independently, who are philosophically in alignment on basic principles like patient centricity and quality care as a fundamental patient right. Two people who have mutual respect, mutual trust and good communication. Admittedly, transformation in healthcare is a daunting task, it is eminently achievable if you have the right number of people to begin, at least two. Anne Marie Benedecto, Vice President, The Joint Commission, gave me sound advice when she said it is ok to think outside the box but our job is much larger—we must "change the box." We are now changing the box at Citrus Valley Health Partners. Our transformation journey continues…

W.T. Choctaw, *Transforming the Patient Experience*,
DOI 10.1007/978-3-319-16928-6_9

Index

W.T. Choctaw, *Transforming the Patient Experience*,
DOI 10.1007/978-3-319-16928-6

Printed in the United States
By Bookmasters